W0106971

Quantitative Assessment in Epilepsy Care

NATO ASI Series

Advanced Science Institutes Series

A series presenting the results of activities sponsored by the NATO Science Committee, which aims at the dissemination of advanced scientific and technological knowledge, with a view to strengthening links between scientific communities.

The series is published by an international board of publishers in conjunction with the NATO Scientific Affairs Division

A	**Life Sciences**	Plenum Publishing Corporation
B	**Physics**	New York and London
C	**Mathematical and Physical Sciences**	Kluwer Academic Publishers
D	**Behavioral and Social Sciences**	Dordrecht, Boston, and London
E	**Applied Sciences**	
F	**Computer and Systems Sciences**	Springer-Verlag
G	**Ecological Sciences**	Berlin, Heidelberg, New York, London,
H	**Cell Biology**	Paris, Tokyo, Hong Kong, and Barcelona
I	**Global Environmental Change**	

Recent Volumes in this Series

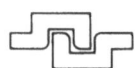

Series A: Life Sciences

Quantitative Assessment in Epilepsy Care

Edited by

Harry Meinardi
Instituut voor Epilepsiebestrijding
Heemstede, The Netherlands

Joyce A. Cramer
Department of Veterans Affairs Medical Center
West Haven, Connecticut, U.S.A.
and Yale University
New Haven, Connecticut, U.S.A.

Gus A. Baker
The Walton Centre
Liverpool, United Kingdom

and

Antonio Martins da Silva
Hospital Geral de Santo António
and Institute of Biomedical Sciences
University of Porto
Porto, Portugal

Springer Science+Business Media, LLC

Proceedings of a NATO Advanced Research Workshop on
Quantitative Assessment in Epilepsy Care,
held April 8–11, 1992,
in Porto, Portugal

NATO-PCO-DATA BASE

The electronic index to the NATO ASI Series provides full bibliographical references (with
keywords and/or abstracts) to more than 30,000 contributions from international scientists
published in all sections of the NATO ASI Series. Access to the NATO-PCO-DATA BASE is
possible in two ways:

—via online FILE 128 (NATO-PCO-DATA BASE) hosted by ESRIN, Via Galileo Galilei,
I-00044 Frascati, Italy

—via CD-ROM "NATO Science and Technology Disk" with user-friendly retrieval software in
English, French, and German (©WTV GmbH and DATAWARE Technologies, Inc. 1989). The
CD-ROM also contains the AGARD Aerospace Database.

The CD-ROM can be ordered through any member of the Board of Publishers or through
NATO-PCO, Overijse, Belgium.

Library of Congress Cataloging-in-Publication Data

Quantitative assessment in epilepsy care / edited by Harry Meinardi ...
  [et al.].
       p.   cm. -- (NATO ASI series. Series A, Life sciences ; vol.
  255)
     "Published in cooperation with NATO Scientific Affairs Division."
     "Proceedings of a NATO Advanced Research Workshop on Quantitative
  Assessment in Epilepsy Care, held April 8-11, 1992, in Porto,
  Portugal"--T.p. verso.
     Includes bibliographical references and indexes.
     ISBN 978-1-4613-6302-6   ISBN 978-1-4615-2990-3 (eBook)
     DOI 10.1007/978-1-4615-2990-3
     1. Epilepsy--Treatment--Standards--Congresses. 2. Epilepsy-
  -Classification--Congresses. 3. Clinimetrics--Congresses.
  4. Epilepsy--Prognosis--Congresses. 5. Health status indicators-
  -Congresses.   I. Meinardi, Harry, 1932-   . II. North Atlantic
  Treaty Organization. Scientific Affairs Division. III. NATO
  Advanced Research Workshop on Quantitative Assessment in Epilepsy
  Care (1992 : Porto, Portugal) IV. Series.
     [DNLM: 1. Epilepsy--classification--congresses. 2. Epilepsy-
  -therapy--congresses. 3. Outcome and Process Assessment (Health
  Care)--congresses. 4. Health Status Indicators--congresses.   WL
  385 Q112 1992]
  RC372.A2Q35   1993
  616.8'5306--dc20
  DNLM/DLC   93-26823
  for Library of Congress   CIP

Additional material to this book can be downloaded from http://extra.springer.com.

ISBN 978-1-4613-6302-6

©1993 Springer Science+Business Media New York
Originally published by Plenum Press, New York in 1993
Softcover reprint of the hardcover 1st edition 1993

All rights reserved

No part of this book may be reproduced, stored in a retrieval system, or transmitted in any
form or by any means, electronic, mechanical, photocopying, microfilming, recording, or
otherwise, without written permission from the Publisher

PREFACE

Advances in epilepsy in recent decades have allowed for improved algorithms for diagnosis and a common understanding of terminology with the development of the International Classifications of Seizures and the Epilepsies. Nevertheless, no common system exists for the estimation of epilepsy severity or its impact on quality of life. Therefore, epileptologists lack the ability to make quantitative assessments of individual patients for comparison of care or for meta-analyses in clinical trials. This book on the Quantitative Assessment of Epilepsy Care approaches this omission by addressing the potential application of clinimetrics within the framework of epilepsy treatment.

Clinimetrics is a fast growing discipline concerned with the quantification of clinical symptoms with respect to decision making relating to diagnosis, treatment, and prognosis. These methods allow for the development and validation of clinical scoring systems. For example, the Glasgow Coma Scale is widely used.

As a chronic disorder, epilepsy would benefit from clinimetric methodology to create uniformity and to allow for comparisons among evaluations. In addition, epileptologists have not yet developed assessments of health related quality of life to define the overall condition of the chronic epilepsy patient and various therapeutic endpoints. While clinimetric tools are essential for research, they will also be useful in clinical practice for the care of individual patients by documenting status and changes over time.

This treatise will provide critical analyses of whether existing rating scales and techniques are valid to use, and which types of scales and techniques require further development.

This is the right time to interpolate aspects of clinimetrics into standard assessments of epilepsy care with the participation of key persons from the international epilepsy community. The International League Against Epilepsy previously introduced world-wide accepted classifications of seizures and of the epilepsies. ILAE is well organized to accept and evaluate the new concept of a clinimetric approach to epilepsy and bring it into general usage.

This volume is the outcome of a workshop held in Porto, Portugal, 8–11 April 1992. An important part of the proceedings is formed by the discussion.

The editors wish to thank the staff of the Serviço de Neurofisiologia, Hospital Geral de Santo Antonio and of the Unit of Human Physiology and Biometrics of the Instituto Ciencias Biomedicas "Abel Salazar," University of Porto, for the excellent conditions created to accomplish the goals of the workshop.

This workshop would not have been possible without the support of NATO. Supplemental financial support from the Netherlands Epilepsy Fund, Marion Merrell Dow, and Wallace Laboratories is gratefully acknowledged.

The editors

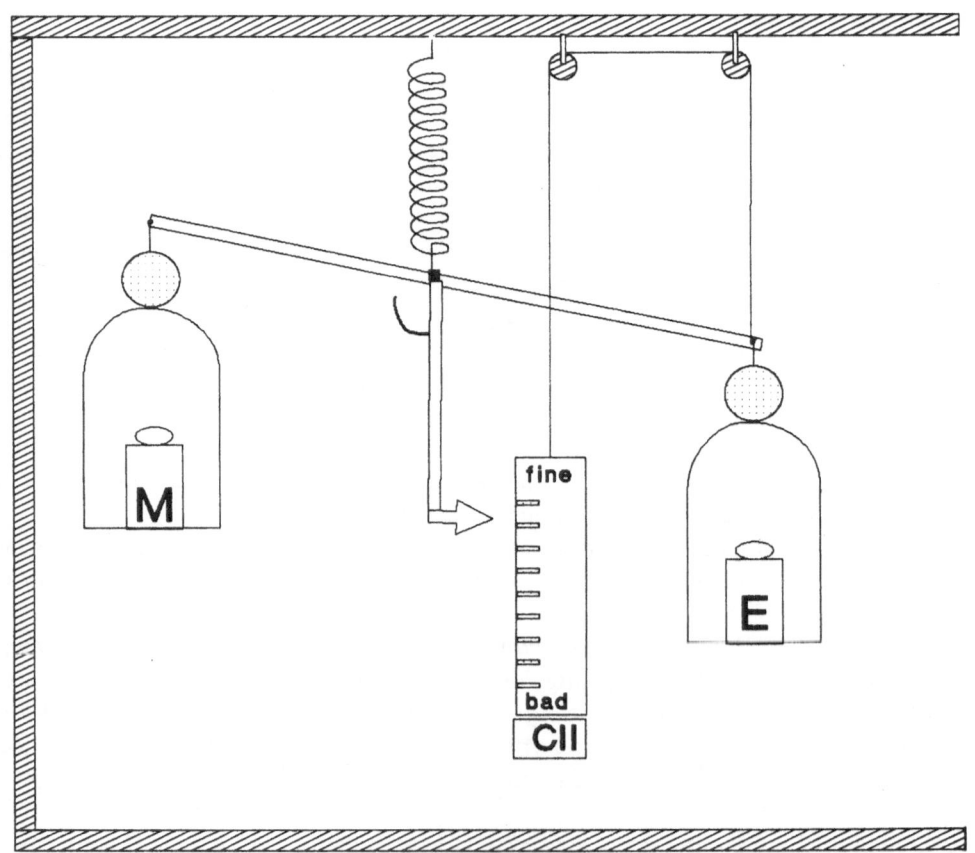

Epilepsy Severity and Control Scales

Clinimetrics deals with scales. The above is a literary example depicting the epileptologist's dilemma: both the severity of the epilepsy [E] and the amount of antiepileptic drug [M] bring the scales to a negative outcome of the Composite Index of Impairment [CII]. Furthermore once the epilepsy is controlled and the scales are in a horizontal position additional medication only leads to a further deterioration of the CII.

CONTENTS

PRINCIPLES AND PRACTICE OF CLINIMETRICS IN EPILEPSY

Alvan R. Feinstein, M.S., M.D.

Sterling Professor of Medicine and Epidemiology
Yale University School of Medicine
New Haven, Connecticut, U.S.A.

CHALLENGES IN MEASUREMENT

The world of clinical medicine offers two different kinds of challenges in measurement. The first kind of challenge, which might be called mensuration, consists of converting the observed phenomena to the basic raw data. Mensuration is what we do when we develop some kind of mechanism and rating scale to express *height* for individual people in **inches or centimetres**, to express *gender* in categories such as **male or female,** or to express *angina pectoris* in categories such as **none, mild, moderate, severe.** *Quantification* is what we do when we take the basic expressions of data for individual people and then form groups of people and expressions that summarize the collected data in each group. Thus, we might form a group of men and express the height of those men in a summary called the *mean*. We might form a group of women and express the proportion of women who have angina itself or the proportion of women who have severe angina. This kind of proportionate occurrence is often called *prevalence*.

We usually express the raw data in classes of information that are called *variables*. The medical variables can contain such demographic features as age, race, and sex. They can also include the things that epidemiologists often call "risk factors," such as smoking, dietary intake, and life style. They can include the information that comes from paraclinical tests such as laboratory procedures, imaging, electroencephalograms, various biopsies and cytologies, and diverse tests of blood, urine, and faeces. Another type of medical variable refers to the identity of different therapeutic agents. There are also the distinctively clinical variables that are obtained from history taking as patients' symptoms and that are noted on physical examination as signs. The clinical variables also include various clinical decisions. There are also diverse kinds of variables that reflect psychic or behavioral status, and other variables that may reflect social status.

Quantitative Assessment in Epilepsy Care, Edited by H. Meinardi et al.
Plenum Press, New York, 1993

PRINCIPLES OF CLINIMETRICS

I use the term *clinimetric indexes*[1] as a name and intellectual home for the rating scales that have been developed for clinical phenomena expressed in specifically clinical data such as history, physical examination, and clinical reasoning. The indexes need not be confined to such data. Some clinimetric indexes can include paraclinical data, but for a rating scale to be called *clinimetric*, it must include at least some clinical phenomena. Examples of reasonably well known clinimetric indexes are the Apgar score, the Jones Diagnostic Criteria for Rheumatic Fever, the Glasgow Coma Scale, the Sickness Impact Profile, the New York Heart Association Functional Categories, and the Karnofsky Performance Index. I also use the word *index* as a generic term for things that are sometimes called indexes, scales, scores, systems, criteria, classes, factors, ratings, and so on.

For example, the Apgar score, developed to describe the clinical condition of a newborn baby, is a well known and well established clinimetric index. Virginia Apgar[2] chose to consider five features of the baby: colour, heart rate, respiration, reflex response to nasal catheter, and muscle tone. She gave each of these five variables a rating score ranging from 0 to 2; and she established criteria for each of those individual ratings, e.g., colour was marked 0 if the baby was blue and pale, 1 if the body was pink but the extremities were blue, and 2 if the baby's colour was all pink. Apgar then arranged to add these five ratings together into a score that ranges from 0 for a dead baby to a 10 for a baby in excellent condition.

I might add that Virginia Apgar was very lucky when she did this work about fifty years ago. She had no consultants to help her. She constructed the index according to her own good common sense; and it is now widely used and valuable throughout the world. I said she was lucky that she had no consultants, because if she had the kind of help that is sometimes given today, she might have produced not the Apgar score, but the Apgar instrument. It would probably be a type of questionnaire containing about 100 items. The first item might be, "I think newborn babies are cute." The respondent would be invited to place a mark or choose a category ranging somewhere from *strongly agree* to *strongly disagree*. The second item might be "When a newborn baby turns blue, I get nervous," with choices from *strongly agree* to *strongly disagree*. The results of the 100-item instrument might have very good statistical scores for the attributes of reliability and validity, but the instrument might not be used at all today because it was too cumbersome and took too long to fill out. Instead, Apgar created the nice, simple score that has been so successful.

Another example of a clinimetric index is the Jones Criteria for the diagnosis of acute rheumatic fever. Dr. T. Duckett Jones[3] developed these criteria about 45 years ago, again without any consultative help. They have also been disseminated, revised several times, and widely used throughout the world. Unlike the Apgar score, however, this index works by forming a cluster of categories rather than a sum of points. Jones identified a set of major manifestations such as carditis, arthritis, chorea, erythema marginatum and subcutaneous nodules. He also identified a set of minor manifestations, such as previous rheumatic fever or heart disease, arthralgia, fever, certain acute phase reactants and a prolonged PR interval. For the cluster of manifestations that allowed diagnosis, the current criteria demand that patients have either two major manifestations or one major and two minor manifestations, plus culture or antibody evidence of a preceding group A streptococcal infection.

The two foregoing examples show that clinical indexes have a general structure beginning with elemental variables such as heart rate or carditis. The elemental variables may be transformed into other scales of expression before the results are aggregated. For example, in the Apgar score, the actual counted heart rate is later transformed into the individual ratings of 0, 1, or 2. The elemental variables may be combined into different axes that form separate subscales. For example, the Jones criteria have a major axis and a minor axis. And then finally, regardless of how the elemental variables or axes are formed, they are aggregated together to form a final or so-called *output scale*. In the Apgar score the output scale ranges from 0 to 10. In the Jones criteria, the output scale has two binary categories: **yes or no**. There may be an additional uncertain rating as well.

Different scales can be used to express the elemental variables of clinical indexes and the output results. The scales can be dimensional for such values as age, height, or weight. They can have ordinal ratings or ranks, such as the graded categories of TNM (Tumor, Nodes, Metastases) stages and the Glasgow coma scale. Things like the Apgar score appear to be quasi-dimensional but they are actually a sum of ordinal ratings for the five constituent scales. Another type of scale that has become popular in recent years is the so-called visual analog scale, in which the patient puts a mark on a line that is usually ten centimetres long with anchors at either end to express the smallest and largest magnitudes of the particular thing being rated. A binary or existential scale reflects the present or absent existence of things like chest pain or dyspnea or an adverse drug reaction or the diagnosis of a disease. Finally, there are nominal scales in which the categories cannot be ranked in any way. Nominal scales might be used for such occupations as **doctor, lawyer, merchant**, etc. or for different categories of religion or for different types of ethnic groups.

Clinimetric indexes can have four main types of function. They can identify status, describe change, make predictions, or serve as guidelines. Status indexes refer to a patient's state at a single point in time. They may be used for the diagnosis of a disease such as rheumatic fever or epilepsy. They can be used to characterize a clinical condition, such as the Apgar score or the Glasgow coma score. They can also be used to identify a therapeutic agent, such as barbiturate, dilantin, etc.

Clinimetric indexes for identifying a change usually refer to a change after treatment. The change can be identified from repeated assessment of single states, for which increments or trends are calculated in the individual measurements. Alternatively, change can be identified from a separate transition index that expresses its ratings in comparative form. For example, a single state index might have categories such as **excellent, good, fair, poor**. A transition scale of categories might be **much better, slightly better, same, slightly worse**, or **much worse**.

Clinimetric indexes have a predictive function when they are used in prognostication. For example, the TNM Staging System for cancer[4] is commonly used to denote the anticipated rates of survival for patients in each stage. And finally, guideline indexes, which are sometimes called clinical algorithms, give instructions or directions for how to do something. Such guidelines have been developed for the activities of nurse practitioners, physicians' associates, or other clinical personnel. Certain guidelines are now being offered (or at times threatened) for activities that might be fiscally compensated in clinical practice.

In the customary principles of evaluation for clinimetric indexes, we basically want to assess accuracy and reproducibility. Because the indexes are contrived rating scales rather than measured dimensions, however, clinicians have often used psychosocial measurement strategies and statistical tests to show what is sometimes called *consistency or reliability or reproducibility*. According to this concept, the index should have good agreement in tests of *intra- and inter-observer variability*. In other words, when applied repeatedly in the same situation, either by the same user or by another user, the index should yield the same results. This type of consistency is usually regarded as a *sine qua non* of scientific measurement.

A second attribute is called *validity*, a term to which psychosocial scientists have prefixed an enormous and often bewildering array of adjectives. The term *criterion validity* represents a check of accuracy against a definitive gold standard measurement. This type of accuracy or criterion validity is regularly available for laboratory measurements where the reference standard might be results obtained at the National Bureau of Standards or at some other laboratory that is generally accepted as doing an excellent job. This type of accuracy can seldom be checked for most clinimetric indexes, however, because a gold standard measurement does not exist. Instead, the psychosocial scientists often look for what they call *construct validity*, which means that they compare the suitability of this index against other indexes that relate to the same phenomenon or against the results that are obtained when the index is applied in actual performance. This type of construct validity is essential when a gold standard is not available. For example, there is no gold standard assessment available for pain. One of the ways in which we might determine, however, that a rating scale for pain has construct validity is to note what I have called "validation by application": the index gives effective results when tested in a contrast of a powerful pain relieving agent versus a placebo.

A particularly important attribute that is sometimes not given full attention in psychosocial strategies and that is absolutely essential for clinimetric indexes, is an attribute I have called *sensibility*, or "clinical common sense." This means that the index must be suitable for its clinical purpose and setting. For example, changes in an electroencephalogram might be accurate and reproducible, but might not be particularly suitable for determining the effects of therapy in patients with epilepsy. The psychometric principle called *face validity* is what we generally mean by clinical common sense.

The attribute of *content validity* refers to the different things that may be included when an index contains many items. For example, in a rating scale for epilepsy, we might include things such as the frequency or severity of attacks, but changes in the patient's weight would not be regarded as a suitable component. We would want the index to have an adequate format of expression. For example if something can be present or absent in different degrees of magnitude, or if we are uncertain about whether it is present or absent, the format of expression would be unsatisfactory if it merely offers a **yes or no** decision. And then finally, we would like the product to be easy to use. The Apgar score, as I indicated earlier, is relatively easy to use, does not take too much time, and is readily understood. The result of a 100-item instrument would not be easy to use and the total sum of ratings might not be particularly clear.

CLINIMETRICS IN EPILEPSY

With that much of a background for clinimetrics in general, we can now turn our attention to clinimetrics in epilepsy. In considering the different functional roles of clinimetric indexes for epilepsy, we are not concerned at this meeting with diagnostic status indexes. We are also not concerned with indexes of prognosis or with developing guideline algorithms for treatment. Our prime concern is in measuring the accomplishment of treatments; and we can therefore begin by considering the conventional targets used in assessing post-therapeutic change.

For remedial therapy, which is intended to improve an existing current state, the target exists when we begin treatment. We can assess progress by directly observing what happens to such targets as pain, dyspnea, or anaemia. With prophylactic therapy, the target is not there when we begin. The goal is to prevent or retard the development of some future state, such as infarction, incapacitation, or death. When a single treatment is aimed at both the remedial and prophylactic goals, the assessment usually requires different indexes. For example, we might remedially want to lower a patient's elevated blood pressure; and the prophylactic goal might be to prevent or retard the development of stroke. Lowering of blood pressure would be assessed with one index, and the occurrence of stroke or other cerebrovascular problems would be measured with some other index. Furthermore, when we measure functional incapacity, the measurement usually reflects the severity of the patient's clinical state. None of these conventional procedures are possible in assessing change for the complexity of epilepsy. One main problem is that epilepsy is not a "state"; it is a condition that occurs in episodes. We therefore need to identify the severity of both the intra-episodic and the inter-episodic events. The measurement cannot be satisfactory if it measures only a single state or changes in a single state. A second problem is that epilepsy, unlike other episodic ailments such as asthma or migraine, can be associated with persistent psychosocial stigmas. A patient's functional incapacity may therefore be a product of psychosocial rather than clinical effects. When a patient is unable to drive a car or unable to work at certain occupations, we may then have "to tease out" the cause as being psychosocial (or occasional legal) constraints, rather than "incapacitation" arising directly from the clinical severity of the ailment itself.

Some of the various attributes that can be assessed for epilepsy are intra-episodic, such as the duration of a particular episode, its severity, and its immediate sequelae. Other attributes are inter-episodic. They reflect the duration of the intervals between episodes, i.e., the frequency of episodes, as well as the patient's functional capacity, or such features as the side effects of therapy.

Among the specific attributes that can be assessed are the characteristics of the seizures themselves. They include the types of manifestations, such as generalized versus focal seizures, tonic or clonic movements, and so on. The severity of these manifestations might be characterized according to the vigour of the clonus, the loss of consciousness, or the magnitude of an injury. The seizures might be associated with predictive features such as an aura, or with a periodic pattern that might be used to modify or prevent the seizures. There can also be a series of precipitating features such as stress, excessive alcohol, sleep deprivation, non-compliance with treatment, or development of an acute co-morbid illness.

There is also, of course, the timing of events with respect to duration and frequency of episodes.

Another set of important attributes for assessment are the consequences of the seizures. They can include the immediate neurologic sequelae, such as aphasia, confusion, tremor and so on. They can also include the persistent sequelae such as affect and mood disturbances, and functional impairment. They would also include the diverse side effects of therapy in oral, cutaneous, neurotoxic, or systemic manifestations.

Among the many problems in forming indexes of assessment, the most obvious first set is to select the attributes to be rated. Which ones will be chosen among the many possibilities, and who makes those choices? Are the choices made by an individual physician, by a committee of experts or other pundits, or by the patient? After those attributes are chosen, the next step is to decide what kind of rating scales will be applied to them. Will they be expressed in binary "existential categories" (such as **yes or no**, **present or absent**), or in ranked ordinal categories, such as **none, mild, moderate, severe**. If an ordinal ranking is chosen, how many categories will be selected?

Alternatively, one can avoid the decisions about number of categories by using a visual analog scale, where the patient puts a mark on a line between various extreme "anchors." If a visual analog scale is chosen, however, what is to be its shape and orientation? Is it a horizontal line, a vertical line, or a curved line? Is it accompanied by anchor labels simply at the two extreme ends, or are additional labels put at intermediate locations? There is no perfect way of making these choices, but different scale-makers will disagree about how to make the choices.

A particularly thorny problem is the combination of attributes. Do we want to preserve all of the individual ratings for all of the individual attributes and then form some method of putting them together, or do we first want to reduce them by forming various groups into so-called *axes* or *subscales*? For example, we might have a rating for each of the individual side effects of therapy in the skin, mouth, and so on. Instead, or in addition, we can establish a separate axis or subscale that offers a single rating for *all* of the side effects. Regardless of whether we keep the individual ratings intact or form them into groups of axes, we then have to decide how to combine the individual or group ratings into a single rating. Will this be done by giving individual scores that are then added to form a sum, or will they be collected into various clusters, such as the tactics that produce various systems with stages ranked as **I, II, III,**...? Alternatively, we can avoid all of these decisions about individual attributes and combinations of attributes by using a single "global" overall rating.

If the individual attributes are preserved, a crucial question is how those attributes should be weighted. Is a batch of three seizures in one day better or worse than having one seizure on each of three days? Is a skin rash more important or less important than problems with the gums? Since these decisions must be made whenever things are combined, a major challenge is the question of how importance is decided. Are the weighing coefficients going to be assigned by a mathematical model? Will they be given a group of arbitrary scores; and if arbitrary scores are given, who makes those decisions?

Any system of measurement, for any clinical condition or state, has to deal with at least four major scientific and statistical challenges. One challenge is that the measurement should be *reproducible*. (This property is sometimes also called *reliability* or *consistency*).

The idea is that the same result should be obtained when the rating is repeated by the same or by another person. The second requirement is that the measurement be *accurate*. This means that the result should agree with the reference value obtained from a so-called "gold-standard" measuring system. The term "validity" is often used for this concept, but because gold-standard measurements are not always available, various "metric mavens" have attached a complex and sometimes bewildering array of adjectives to the word "validity," for use when accuracy cannot be measured. A third important requirement might be called *sensibility*. It is also sometimes called *face validity*. The idea here is that the result should make good clinical common sense in demonstrating what we really want to know. Finally, another requirement has more recently been called *responsiveness*. It refers to whether repeated measurements will discern the change that we want to show.

In the management of the foregoing four challenges, consistency or reproducibility is usually to difficult to test for epilepsy. We can try to get the same person—who might be either a patient or a clinician—to repeat the rating, but we can seldom assemble different patients and clinicians for examinations that will be conducted at the same place and time. In the assessment of accuracy for epilepsy, no "gold standards" are available. Various objective measurements in laboratory data or electroencephalograms might be quite accurate, but they seldom measure the most important entities to be considered, and besides, their measurement will often distract attention from the proper focus on what is happening to the patient and to the patient's life.

With respect to *sensibility*, there is a divergency of opinions, in epilepsy as well as in any other clinical measurement, about what approach "makes sense," what attributes to include in the measurement, and how to assign weights to those attributes. For dealing with *responsiveness*, two guidelines are readily apparent about what to avoid. The first is try *not* to use what might be called a "mega-variable" index, having a large number of constituent variables or "items." The added combination of all those results may obscure important changes in the main variable that we want to know about. The second thing to be avoided is an oligo-category rating scale, having very few categories, such as four or fewer. In this situation, the individual "coarse" categories may not be sensitive enough to discern change within the same category.

CONCLUSIONS AND RECOMMENDATIONS

In preparation for this conference, I was sent copies of pertinent indexes that had been prepared and presented in excellent papers by Cramer et al[5], by Duncan and Sander[6], and by Wijsman et al[7]. The Cramer paper also has a brief outline of four additional rating scales. Each of the seven approaches has its own abundant merits; but the total group, when examined collectively, offers a splendid illustration of the problems I have been discussing. The authors have chosen different attributes to be included in each index; they have given different weights to the individual components; they have combined the weighted components in different ways; and they have used the indexes in different manners for assessing change.

If you have any hope of attaining consensus in the deliberations at this workshop, I would suggest that the problems to be resolved be divided into four specific sources of disagreement: attributes, scales, combinatory methods, and weights. You can then focus your intellectual and disputatious energies on trying to identify the specific things that you disagree about within these sources. After you have clearly identified your disagreements, you can then determine how to resolve them.

In my own clinimetric adventures, I have found that investigators often argue vigorously, without any progress being attained, because they have not clearly circumscribed the domain of each type of disagreement. They are then unable to focus clearly on what needs to be done. I therefore urge you to consider that your disagreements can arise: from the particular topics or attributes to be considered in each index; from the scales you choose to express them; from the ratings of importance to be assigned to each topic; from the way you combine the different topics to form a single final rating; and finally, from the measurement of change itself.

I should like to offer a few recommendations about which you might want immediately to agree or disagree before you begin working on your other disagreements. I would urge you, above all, to concentrate on issues of sensibility and responsiveness, avoiding the current statistical infatuation with an index's reliability and validity. The statistical approaches are splendid as acts of statistics, but they often do not produce good clinical sense and they are often not effective in patient care. If you are worried about reliability, but are not easily able to test for it, make sure that the directions for the index are clearly stated so that the process can be readily understood and repeated. Keep in mind that some of the most important indexes used in patient care today—particularly things like the Apgar score and the TNM staging system for cancer—have never been subjected (as far as I know) to any test of reliability. Nevertheless, their usage is quite clear and their results have been invaluable in clinical medicine. A second recommendation I would make is that instead of fighting about how to rate importance, let the patient—rather than various experts, pundits, or mathematical models—decide what is important to include and how to weight it. It is the patient who has the epilepsy; it is the patient whose life is being affected by treatment; and it is the patient who ought to decide what is important and what constitutes a good result of treatment.

To let patients indicate importance while still arriving at some kind of standardized score, I have recently been doing some research with a colleague, Dr. James Wright, an orthopaedic surgeon, on rating scales for patient's status before hip replacement. We have used the following approach: First, let the patient (or perhaps a clinician,) rate the magnitude or severity of each selected attribute. For epilepsy, you can rate the magnitude of severity for such attributes as injury, incontinence, duration of seizures, frequency, occurrence of diverse forms of neurotoxicity, etc. Next, let the *patient* rate the importance of each attribute that has been cited. For this purpose, patients can use a visual analog scale or a category scale to indicate whether they regard the particular attribute as having no, very little, or very substantial importance. Next, form a severity-importance rating for each attribute as the product obtained by multiplying the two ratings for severity and importance. Then take the sum of the severity-importance ratings for all the attributes. This sum will produce what might be called a "severity-importance score." The next step is to determine what the maximum severity-importance score might be for each patient. For this purpose, take the worst severity rating that could be given for each of the particular attributes; multiply it by the patient's importance rating for each attribute; and take their sum. The *patient-specific* score is then standardized as the ratio of the two sums. It emerges when the sum of each the patient's severity-importance ratings is divided by the patient's maximum possible rating.

This ratio will range from 0–1, but it can be multiplied by 100 to yield a score that ranges from 0, which is the best situation, to 100, which is the worst. The rating is specific for each patient because the patient chooses the importance of each attribute. The rating is standardized because it is expressed on a scale of 0 to 1 or 0 to 100. You can then repeat these ratings at diverse intervals and compare the patient's successive scores to see what kind of progress is being made. The numbers themselves will be standardized; but their the contents will reflect the patient's particular observations, aspirations, and goals.

As an alternative or additional approach that is much simpler, you can try to let the patient give a "global" rating of improvement. In this situation, the patient expresses a rating on a single global scale—it can contain categories or a visual-analog format. The patient marks the degree of improvement with a simple, single rating. Such ratings are not scientifically appealing because the constituent elements are not identified. Nevertheless, the approach is highly sensible and it avoids the imposition of any arbitrary weights produced by outsiders. It also corresponds to probably the most well known and traditional clinical question used in medicine: "How are you?". After getting the how-are-you and how-have-you-changed ratings, you can always add extra questions if you want to get the patient's specifications for what has improved. This tactic may appear to be scientifically primitive and psychometrically repugnant, but the approach has regularly been found—by the Food and Drug Administration of the United States and by many data analysts—to be the most powerful index of "efficacy" for therapy; and the simple global ratings have often been used as a "gold standard" for validating the components of other rating systems.

In an era of major concern about the decline of humanism in medicine and about the lack of attention to patients rather than to technologic devices and therapy, I would point out that highly complex systems of measurement are often analogous to other types of technology. The results may be scientifically magnificent, but the patient is often neglected during the process. The resurrection of attention, respect, and quantification for the question, "How are you?," may be a highly effective way to deal with some of our current challenges in science, clinimetric measurement, and humanism.

REFERENCES

1. Feinstein, A.R. Clinimetrics. New Haven. Yale University Press. 1987.
2. Apgar, Virginia. A proposal for a new method of evaluation of the newborn infant. Anesth Analg 1953; 32:260–7.
3. Jones, T.D. The diagnosis of rheumatic fever. JAMA 1944; 126:481.
4. American Joint Committee for Cancer Staging and End Results Reporting. Manual for staging of cancer. Chicago, 1977.
5. Cramer, J.A., Smith D.B., Mattson R.H., et al. A method of quantification for the evaluation of antiepileptic drug therapy. Neurology 1983; 33:26–37.

6. Duncan, J.S., Sander J.W.A.S. The Chalfont Seizure Severity Scale. J Neurol Neurosurg Psychiatry 1991; 54:873–876.
7. Wijsman, D.J.P., Hekster, Y.A., Renier, W.O., Meinardi, H. Clinimetrics and epilepsy care. Pharm Weekbl [Sci] 1991; 13:182–188.

STATISTICAL ASPECTS OF THE MEASUREMENT
OF CLINICAL CARE IN EPILEPSY

A L Johnson, PhD, CStat

Medical Statistician
Medical Research Council Biostatistics Unit
Institute of Public Health
University Forvie Site
Cambridge CB2 2SR
United Kingdom

INTRODUCTION

From the viewpoint of a physician epilepsy is a complex chronic disease which manifests as a "recurrent paroxysmal disorder of cerebral function characterised by sudden, brief attacks of altered consciousness, motor activity, or sensory phenomena" (Taber 1985). The definition though terse encapsulates the essential features of epilepsy and hints at the heterogeneity of the disorder especially with the "catch-all" term "sensory phenomena." From the viewpoint of a statistician the disease manifests as a sequence of disjoint and perhaps heterogeneous episodes of variable, but comparatively short duration, distributed non-randomly over an extended period of observation. The episodes may be clustered in groups, confined to an early epoch in the period of observation, absent for long intervals, or perhaps recurrent and frequent throughout the whole period of observation. Given such a rich variety of patterns for seizure recurrence it is not surprising that numerous measures have been employed both to portray the progression of epilepsy over time, and to summarise and assess the comparative usefulness of treatment. These in turn have led to diverse methods of statistical analysis from the simplest summary statistics and two group comparisons to the more complicated repeated measures analysis of variance, and regression modelling techniques for "survival" type data.

The aim of this paper is to review, from a statistical viewpoint, some of the measures for quantitative assessment of epilepsy which have been employed in the past, to comment on their validity, usefulness, analysis and summarisation, and to consider whether or not, they may be combined into scales which measure the severity of epilepsy and quality of life. Attention is also drawn to recent developments in statistical modelling techniques

Quantitative Assessment in Epilepsy Care, Edited by H. Meinardi et al.
Plenum Press, New York, 1993

which may help to provide a better framework for exploring and understanding the complex presentation of epilepsy.

SEIZURE FREQUENCY AND SEIZURE COUNTS

With a disease which manifests as a series of recurrent episodes it is natural perhaps to summarise the course in terms of seizure frequency, or number of seizures per unit of time. Indeed like classification such a measure is ubiquitous throughout comparative studies of the efficacy of AED's (Coatsworth 1971). Seizure counts and frequencies may be analyzed and summarised using statistical methods for handling continuous variables; sometimes they are reduced by grouping (or splitting) to ordered categorical (or binary) data. The estimation and interpretation of seizure frequencies is not as straight-forward as would appear, and some care is necessary to ensure that meaningful conclusions are drawn from appropriate analyses. There are several important points to bear in mind, and it is useful to remember that a frequency has two components, namely a count which forms the numerator, and a time interval which forms the denominator. In the numerator we need an accurate count of (all) seizures, which is perhaps relatively simple for major tonic-clonic episodes, but considerably more difficult when counting partial seizures or myoclonic jerks especially since these tend to cluster, and may take place over an extended interval; in status-epilepticus the boundary between successive seizures may not be discernible.

In patients who suffer frequent seizures the counting will need to be done by an observer; in the community it is necessary to rely on information supplied by the patient, perhaps aided by a seizure diary. Precise dating of seizures is not strictly necessary. In the denominator we need a specified period defined first by a reference starting point and secondly, by an interval. For example, in a clinical trial the starting point would be the date of randomisation, or another date at a defined interval after it; in an observational study it would be related to a specific event such as an index seizure as in the National General Practice Study of Epilepsy (Hart et al 1990). The duration of the actual period over which seizures are counted depends on the nature of the patient sample and the objectives of the study.

Great care must be taken when estimating seizure frequencies over periods of differing duration in different patients. The problem is illustrated in Figure 1, which shows a decline in the risk of seizures over time from the start of therapy. The two patients exhibit

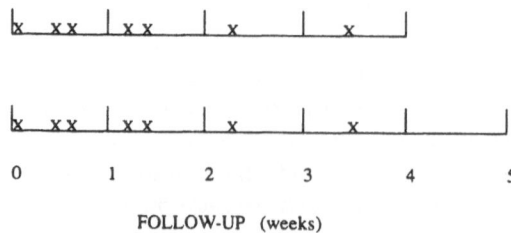

FOLLOW-UP (weeks)

Figure 1. Seizure recurrence in two patients.

similar seizure frequencies over the initial 4 weeks of observation (namely 1.75 seizures per week), but will give different frequencies (1.75 and 1.40 seizures per week respectively) if the complete observation period for the second patient is used in the denominator. This suggests that frequencies should be estimated over similar periods in all patients, and that variable periods of observation should not be used, except in the rare cases where it is safe to assume that risk of seizure recurrence does not vary with time.

The summarisation of frequencies also requires considerable care. Summary statistics must convey useful information about the underlying distribution. In many papers seizure frequencies are summarised by means (and standard deviations (SD)) and it is not unusual to find estimates of the form 4.3 (2.9) seizures per month, for example. A little thought can discern the misleading nature of such a statement. We know that about 95% of frequencies will lie within 2SD's of the mean for data that are Normally distributed, so the summary statement above tells us that approximately 95% of frequencies in the sampled population lie between 4.3 − 2 × 2.9 and 4.3 + 2 × 2.9, that is −1.5 and 10.1 seizures per month. Since seizure frequencies cannot be negative the summary statistics convey no useful information, except that the distribution of frequencies is highly skewed. Use of the standard error (SE) does not alleviate this problem although it may beguile the unwary; a mean seizure frequency (SE) of 10 (2.3) seizures per year looks more sensible, but if we know that the sample size is 100, we can estimate the SD as 10 × 2.3, or 23 seizures per year, and we are back with the same problem. We are attempting to summarise seizure frequencies on an inappropriate scale, and instead we need to find a way of coping with the skewed distribution and of providing meaningful summaries. Some authors are aware of the problem especially in the context of clinical trials where the objective is to compare changes in seizure frequency (treatment period minus baseline period), among different treatment groups. Faced with data that exhibit wide variation (and perhaps no statistically significant differences) the seizure counts are reduced to percentage changes, which are then dichotomised below and above 50%. The result is the familiar reporting of differences between percentages of patients who exhibit at least a 50% reduction in seizures over the baseline. Apart from a change from 500 to 250 seizures per year in one patient being regarded as equivalent to that from 4 to 2 in another, and the selection of a rather arbitrary cut-off point (50%), the comparative measure of efficacy is rather remote from the raw data, the seizure counts, and requires some mental agility to understand what it actually means. There are several alternatives, which should be considered instead, before the use of such drastic data reduction. In general it is useful to select summary statistics which are as close as possible to the data themselves. The choice should be based on experience of analyzing similar data, and on exploratory analyses.

First it is useful to report the median seizure frequency in the sample (this is the 50th centile); addition of the 25th and 75th centiles will provide some idea of spread. Occasionally it will be possible to report means as well, but only in samples of patients who exhibit a consistent seizure recurrence pattern. Skewed distributions arise from samples which include patients who have no seizures at all, as well as those with some patients who have very high seizure frequencies. For the former it is appropriate to report the percentage of patients who are seizure-free, as well as the median (25th, 75th centiles) in those who are not; for the latter it is useful to ascertain whether there is a fairly continu-

Table 1. Seizure counts over 12 weeks from a crossover trial of Lamotrigine and Placebo as add-on therapy in refractory epilepsy

	Period 1		Period 2	
	Lamotrigine	Placebo	Lamotrigine	Placebo
(Number of patients)	(10)	(11)	(11)	(10)
Median	20.5	27.0	13.0	49.5
Mean	21.6	36.7	15.9	70.0
SD	13.7	24.0	12.4	58.2

(SD - Standard Deviation)

ous spread of seizure counts, or just one or two extreme observations, which may be regarded as outliers.

Secondly it is informative to examine the distribution of frequencies, and to investigate whether or not, transformation of the data may be helpful. In clinical trials frequencies are often estimated from seizure counts over a standard period, so we may work directly with the counts themselves. Since counts of recurrent events tend to follow a Poisson distribution we may try transforming the counts by taking square roots (maybe after first adding one). Of course the square root of seizure counts is not a natural scale which is readily interpretable to either physician or patient, so summary statistics will need to be back-transformed. A related transformation, taking logarithms (again perhaps after the addition of one, so as to avoid zeros), may provide both reasonable analysis and interpretation. Here back-transformation provides an estimate of proportional change. The assumptions which underlie any method of statistical analysis should be understood, and verified for the data to which they are applied. Assumptions of Normality can be checked using diagnostic plots and test statistics (Altman 1991). Samples with seizure frequencies clumped at both extremes, and others which generate awkward distributions, may require aggregation of the individual frequencies into groups, with analysis by methods appropriate for ordered categorical data (Agresti 1990). Arbitrary dichotomisation should be avoided.

Seizure counts are particularly popular measures of outcome in phase 2 and early phase 3 crossover trials in patients with intractable epilepsy, where a new AED and either a standard AED or placebo, are added randomly to existing therapy. Such patients usually have recurrent seizures over an interval of 2 or 3 months, and there is some hope that if a new AED is effective, then this can be demonstrated with a comparatively small number of patients. Jones and Kenward (1989) provide an excellent detailed background to the analysis of crossover trials, including some diagnostic plots to check that the assumption of Normally distributed random errors (or residuals) is reasonable.

As an example we take seizure counts over two 12 week periods from a randomised crossover trial of Lamotrigine and placebo as add-on therapy in 21 patients with refractory seizures, conducted in Cardiff (Jawad et al 1989). Table 1 shows some summary statistics for the two treatment groups in each period. The inappropriateness of the means and standard deviations is immediately apparent for the reasons given above. Also we can see that there is some divergence between the means and medians, indicating skewed distributions of counts; that the medians are lower than the means suggests that the skew arises from high counts in some patients.

Further, as shown in Figure 2 the SD's increase almost linearly with the means suggesting logarithmic transformation (the plot of log(SD) against log(mean) is linear with slope only slightly larger than one). Analysis on the log-scale, followed by back-transformation suggests a 60% (95% confidence limits (CL): 41% and 73%) reduction in seizures on average with Lamotrigine compared with placebo; a rather more useful summary than recording that 18 of 21 patients had fewer seizures on Lamotrigine than on placebo (so seizure reduction in 86% (95% CL: 63%, 97%)), or that 14 patients had at least a 50% reduction in seizure frequency while taking Lamotrigine compared with the frequency while taking placebo (50% reduction in 67% (43%,85%)).

So far we have concentrated on counting seizures of all types. However seizure counts may be delineated by type whenever the data allow. Indeed it is not unusual to encounter separate analyses of counts of partial seizures and tonic-clonic seizures. The remarks above apply to these analyses as well. Finally it is pertinent to echo the remark that to count seizures properly patients need to be followed over the full period of intended observation. Interpolation from a restricted to a longer period may produce the problem highlighted in Figure 1. With incomplete counts it is wise to subdivide the whole follow-

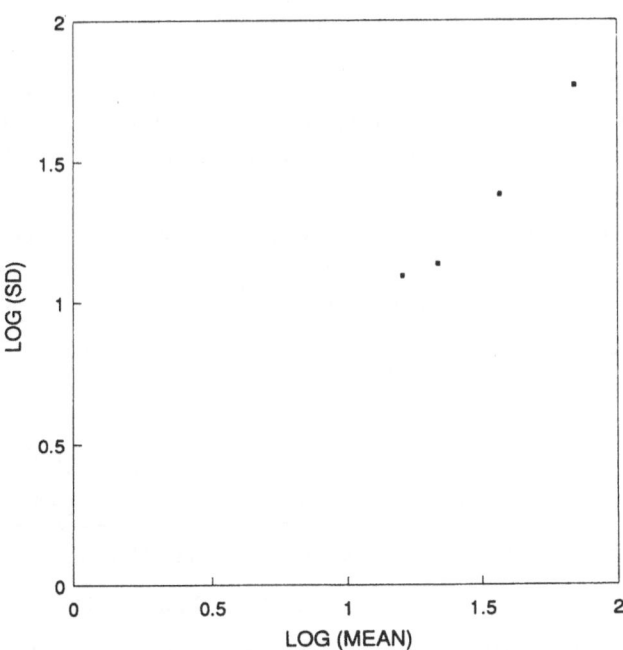

Figure 2. Crossover trial seizure counts.

up period into sub-intervals, and either conduct the analyses within these sub-periods, or use a statistical model to estimate the missing sub-period counts, which may then be aggregated.

SEIZURE-FREE PERIOD

While seizure counts may help to quantify disease progression in patients with resistant or intractable seizures, they are not a useful quantifier in the great majority of people with epilepsy, who reside in the community, and either do not have "active" epilepsy (Goodridge and Shorvon 1983), or suffer only infrequent seizures. Counting seizures in such patients usually means waiting a long period of time. Instead it is quite common to focus on the proportion (or percentage) of patients who remain seizure-free at specified intervals from a nominated date, which again may be the date of randomisation in a clinical trial, or a registration date in an observational study. Percentages of patients who are seizure-free, say at 1 year from the nominated date have been estimated in a variety of ways, all of which may be labelled (technically) as crude.

Table 2 shows some of these crude estimates against the background of a (fictitious) study with 100 patients, 10% of whom are followed for less than a year; the estimates vary according to how the patients followed for less than one year are accounted for: the first two use the number known seizure-free at 1 year divided by the total in the sample (a), and the total followed for 1 year (b); the last two estimate the risk of seizure recurrence from the total sample (c), and from the total of those followed for 1 year or with seizure recurrence (d). If all patients had been followed for one year, then the crude estimates would all be the same, which may be seen as a persuasive argument for intensive follow-up. However this ignores practicalities, for patients are enroled into studies over an extended interval and some will be followed for a shorter period, not because of loss, but simply because insufficient time has elapsed. The crude estimates should not be used. The solution is to adopt an actuarial (life-table or Kaplan-Meier) estimator which can take account of varying follow-up

Table 2. Some crude estimates of percentage seizure-free at one year

Follow-up Time	Status at 1 year or last follow-up < 1 year		
	Seizure-free	Seizure	Total
< 1 year	n_{1f} (5)	n_{1s} (5)	n_1 (10)
> 1 year	n_{2f} (25)	n_{2s} (65)	n_2 (90)
Total	n_f (30)	n_s (70)	n (100)

(Numbers in brackets are for illustration based on sample of 100 patients)

(a) $100 \times n_{2f}/n = 25.0\%$

(b) $100 \times n_{2f}/n_2 = 27.8\%$

(c) $100 \times (1 - n_s/n) = 30.0\%$

(d) $100 \times \{1 - n_s/(n_s + n_{2f})\} = 26.3\%$

times. For the life-table estimate the follow-up period is divided into contiguous sub-periods and the risk of recurrence within each is calculated as the number of patients who have their first seizure recurrence within the sub-period, divided by the total number of patients still seizure-free at the start of the sub-period minus half the number of these patients who are not followed to the end of the sub-period; this estimate is subtracted from one to give the proportion seizure-free (in Table 2 the estimate is 1-(70/95), or 26.3%). The proportions seizure-free in each sub-period are multiplied together to obtain the actuarial estimate of the proportion seizure-free at each stage of follow-up. The alternative Kaplan-Meier estimate uses the exact interval from the starting date to the date of seizure recurrence, or the last date of follow-up in those who remain seizure-free. A detailed and readable account of actuarial techniques can be found in Peto et al (1976, 1977).

An example from epilepsy is contained in the report of the Medical Research Council anti-epileptic drug withdrawal trial (AEDWS), (Medical Research Council Antiepileptic Drug Withdrawal Study Group 1991), where the figure shows the percentages of patients remaining seizure-free up to 5 years from randomisation to the two treatment policies; it also indicates the numbers of patients at risk of recurrence and the hazard rates and ratio during follow-up. Such summaries are more informative than crude estimates at one or two arbitrarily chosen intervals.

It is usual to plot the percentages seizure-free from seizures of all types, perhaps because sample sizes are inadequate to allow finer sub-division. In principle, however there is no reason why actuarial analyses should not present percentages free of tonic-clonic seizures, or of some other specific seizure type. Other modifications are also possible, for example, in clinical trials where the initial risk of seizure recurrence may depend upon initial dose of AED, seizures occurring in a titration period (perhaps the first three months) may be ignored.

Actuarial methods are applicable to studies with prolonged observation of patients which require follow-up to a defined endpoint; in this section we have concentrated on one defined as the first seizure after a specified starting date. Alternatively, we could have nominated the second, or the tenth seizure, or perhaps the fifth day on which a seizure occurred. The choice is left to the investigator and obviously should be clinically useful. Actuarial methods really require fairly precise dating of seizures, and this is not always straight-forward. When exact dates are available, they should be used (which still leaves the problem of deciding how to distinguish multiple seizures on the same day when interest centres on the second or subsequent seizure). If exact dates are not known then interpolation may be necessary. There are no guidelines for this; the obvious and most practical is to assume that seizures are equally spaced; so with "approx 6 seizures from March to end of July," an interval of 153 days, we assume a seizure every 21.9 days, or 22 March, 13 April, 5 May, 26 May, 17 June, and 9 July.

REMISSION FROM SEIZURES

The objective of AED therapy is to prevent seizure recurrence, not just in the short-term, but over extended intervals. Achievement of such periods of remission not only allows patients with a history of epilepsy to lead comparatively normal lives in the community, but may also suggest the possibility of AED withdrawal. Whereas the interval from a nominated starting date to (first) seizure recurrence concentrates on the rather negative aspect of epilepsy, as well as on an event which usually occurs within a comparatively short term, the interval to achievement of remission focuses on a more positive aspect and longer term outcome.

Of course, the choice of the period of remission is somewhat arbitrary, but it should be pragmatic (reasonable numbers of patients achieve it), as well as meaningful. Obvious choices are 1 and 2 years in prospective studies (the latter corresponding to the interval for (re-)application for a driving licence in UK and some other European countries). Periods longer than this are not used because of practical difficulties in following patients over many years; however 5 years remission has been used in a retrospective study (Annegers et al 1979). An example using two-year remission in a randomised clinical trial of phenytoin and sodium valproate is presented by Turnbull et al (1985).

The estimation of the cumulative percentage of patients achieving a specified remission period is again made using actuarial techniques. For example, with 1 year remission, the interval from the starting date to completion of the first full year of follow-up without seizures is the "event of interest." When seizure dates are not known precisely, they should be interpolated (see above). Calculation is easiest when based on calendar year (rather than the "exact" year of 365.25 days). Thus a patient with successive (interpolated) seizures on 1 April in two successive years does not achieve a one year remission, while another patient with seizures only on 1 April one year and 2 April in the successive year does. Just as for seizure-free period, time to remission may be restricted to specific seizure types.

AED DOSAGE

The prescribed dose of an AED is readily recorded. Unfortunately it cannot be used as a quantifier of care since the dose of AED actually taken is subject to massive measurement error.

AED SERUM CONCENTRATIONS

Assays for the concentrations of the major AED's in serum have been available for 20 years, and are now routine in the everyday management of patients with epilepsy. To some extent they subvert the problem of dose monitoring by at least indicating whether or not a patient is actually taking the drug prescribed. However as a result of the complex pharmacokinetics of some AED's, they are a poor guide to actual dosage consumed. Serum concentrations are "almost" continuous, though over a limited range, statistically a mixture distribution. One component of the mixture is the patients not taking the AED, or who have undetectable serum levels (summarised as a percentage of all patients); the other is the patients who have concentrations from the minimum detectable to the maximum tolerated (summarised by 25th, 50th and 75th centiles, together with minimum and maximum).

ADVERSE SIDE EFFECTS

It is well documented that AED's cause adverse side-effects both in children and adults. Although their incidence is usually reported in comparative studies of AED's, they often appear of secondary importance, with the primary analysis focusing on seizure prevention. If there is little to choose between the efficacy of the major AED's, then adverse side effects become of paramount importance since their nature and severity will determine the choice of AED for a particular patient. Each adverse effect is usually recorded as a binary variable (absent/present), except perhaps biochemical and haematological variables for which actual concentrations are noted; however the latter are usually simplified and presented either as below, within, or above some comparative (normal) range, or perhaps below or above a critical cut-off point.

The incidence of side-effects is usually summarised in one or two of a variety of (fairly elementary) ways: percentages (proportions) of patients who report any, at least one of a designated list, each or at least one of a specific group, critical events and so on. Side-effects may be aggregated and reported as a distribution of number per patient. Sometimes percentages of occasions (such as clinic visits) when adverse effects have been noted, are presented.

Adverse side-effects also highlight the need to look at outcome measures in different ways for each may pick-up different aspects of treatment. For example, in a clinical trial of two AED's, we may discover only minor differences in the overall incidence of side-effects (perhaps a median of 1.2 per patient on one treatment, compared with 1.3 per patient on the other, after 8 weeks), and consequently no overall preference for one treatment policy on this measure of outcome. However, if the side-effects are treatment-specific (as hirsutism with phenytoin, or weight-gain with sodium valproate) there will certainly be preferences for specific patients, and analysis of an aggregated score alone will hide these.

Whereas considerable effort is often devoted to the analysis of seizure counts and frequencies, sometimes using multivariate regression techniques to adjust comparative treatment effects for important prognostic variables, the analysis of adverse side effects is reduced to a much more mundane level. This may be justified, or it may stem from lack of appreciation that the requisite techniques are also available for binary variables in the form of logistic regression analysis (Hosmer and Lemeshow 1989), which is also fully implemented in the more popular computer packages. An elegant and simple account has been written by Fleiss et al (1986).

COMBINING MEASURES

Up to this point we have considered the most popular measures which are used to characterise epilepsy, its prognosis and treatment. Each of these dimensions has been examined individually and there has been no attempt to amalgamate or trade-off one with another. There are two principal reasons for this; first these measures are usually presented in this way, and secondly this form of summarisation is very close to the raw data, and consequently comparatively easy to understand and interpret. In addition we know sufficient about the distribution of patients on these measures, to enable their use in sample size calculations during the design stage of clinical trials, or epidemiological studies. We need very good reasons indeed for wandering too far from the basic measurements themselves. It must be stressed that when several measures are to be combined into one, it is vital that the statistical properties (especially the distributions) of each of the individual component measures are well understood; combining inappropriate summary statistics on several measures does not yield a useful or valid scale. As shown in some of the previous sections there are still misunderstandings about how to summarise some of the basic measures themselves.The sections which follow refer briefly to scales for assessing severity of epilepsy, indicate the key steps in constructing a rating scale, and discuss a few ways in which two or more dimensions may be combined in the same analysis.

RATING SCALES FOR SEIZURE SEVERITY

There have been suggestions that merely counting seizures does not provide an adequate measure of either the severity of epilepsy, or the outcome of treatment (Cramer et al 1983; Duncan and Sander 1991). One result has been the recent construction of rating scales which assign scores on various dimensions of the disease and its treatment, and then aggregate over them to derive a global measure (Cramer et al. 1983, Duncan and Sander 1991, Baker GA et al. 1991). The scales are described and discussed elsewhere in this volume.

In counting seizures we are doing exactly that, and whether or not the total is a surrogate for seizure severity is a separate issue; counts of similar items we do understand, we can analyze and interpret. However since seizures manifest in a variety of forms one question is whether or not we should regard them all as roughly equivalent, and simply count across all types (like a rating scale which assigns weights of one to all items), or move to the other extreme and regard one type of over-riding importance (a rating scale with all weights except one equal to zero).

Gordon et al (1988) point out that a concept has reached the stage of measurement research when it can be defined operationally, there is a specifiable technique for measuring it, and there is agreement on the outcomes of measurement. It is apparent from papers and discussions at this workshop, that while there is broad agreement that a scale for measuring seizure severity is required, there is no clear clinical consensus about how to compose it. The scales that have been developed contain some common core features, and these could serve as a starting point.

However there are some fundamental issues which require resolution. First the measurement of seizure severity is inappropriate in patients who are seizure-free, as well as in those patients who exhibit a very low seizure frequency; but where is the threshold, and is it dependent upon seizure type? For patients in the community who do not suffer frequent seizures, and indeed may experience long periods in remission, it may be the occurrence of a seizure and its psychosocial consequences which are important. Secondly in patients who exhibit a high seizure frequency (and certainly those in whom the number of seizures is uncountable), a measure of seizure severity independent of frequency may be useful; again, where is the threshold? Finally since the majority of patients have seizures of just one type, should a measure of severity be type dependent? Seizure severity scales will perhaps find most frequent usage in the setting of hospital based studies with patients who suffer regular seizures; how much they will add to the study of seizure frequency alone, requires detailed investigation.

RATING SCALES IN GENERAL

The purpose of this section is to provide a path for the construction of a rating scale from its conception to its actual use, by highlighting some of the more important stages of development. There is now a substantial literature actually dealing with the construction of rating scales, and for assessing their properties. Readers are referred to Feinstein 1987; van Knippenberg and de Haes 1988; Gordon 1988; Morley and Snaith 1989; Streiner and Norman 1989 and Thompson 1989 for a detailed discussion of the points presented here.

In the following the term rating scale is used as a synonym for rating index, rating instrument or schedule, and consists of (subscale) measures on one or more separate dimensions (or facets); these in turn are each assessed by one or more component items. The simplest form of rating scale thus consists of just one item on a single dimension (in effect a single variable); an intermediate has single items on separate dimensions; and the most complex has multiple subscales composed of multiple items. Of course, each sub-scale can, and should be treated as a separate rating scale, but when subscale scores are to be combined a global perspective is also required.

A. Objectives

(1) establish the purpose of the scale with an overall idea of what it is intended to record, and over what period of time.

(2) establish the broad characteristics of the population of people who are expected to provide the information recorded by the scale (whether self-rated or obtained by an independent observer), and check that the purpose of the scale is relevant to them.

B. Equivalence

(1) ascertain whether there is already a suitable scale in existence, or one which can be adapted to the required purposes.

(2) consider whether a single global question (perhaps in the form of an analogue scale) will suffice instead of a multi-item rating instrument, especially bearing in mind that it may be given to the same patient several times.

C. Dimensions

(1) agree by consensus the dimensions or facets, which it is necessary to evaluate in order to meet the purposes for which the scale is required (content validity). Without

a gold standard there is no formal method to check this, and the only recourse is to extended discussion and wide consultation.

(2) ascertain whether there are existing scales, or single items (variables or analogue scales) to measure any of these individual dimensions.

D. Items

(1) agree by consensus the component items for each dimension.

(2) decide how each item will be recorded and rated; either as a binary (yes/no) variable, or an ordered categorical variable perhaps on a 3, 4 or 5 point Likert scale, or a continuous variable.

(3) check that the meaning of each item is clear and understood.

(4) decide how the items on a single dimension will be combined to yield a score on that dimension. These vary from very simple methods, such as addition, and hierarchical scoring to very complicated algorithms. In general the simplest are best, unless there are explicit reasons for more complex systems. (The problems of assigning weights have been discussed recently in an important paper by Cox et al (1992); they recommend avoidance of explicit weighting schemes, the use of simple schemes, and ultimately sensitivity analyses, and checks on robustness of conclusions to alternative, arbitrary choices of weights).

(5) decide whether the scores on the separate subscales will be aggregated, and if so how.

Sections (E) to (G) apply to each subscale or dimension whether this is a single variable or an aggregation over several items, as well as to the aggregated score over subscales.

E. Development

(1) build up profiles of archetypal patients or subjects, who are envisaged as falling towards the two extremes of the scale, and at one or two intermediate points along it;

(2) apply the subscale to them and examine their scores in relationship to the extreme points (theoretical minimum and maximum). The aim is to ensure that the scale is sensibly structured. If the extreme archetypes are remote from the theoretical limits of the scale, some restructuring may be advised. Check that the intermediate archetypes lie at sensible intervals between the extremes.

F. Structure

(1) obtain item ratings and dimension scores for a heterogeneous sample of subjects and examine the responses to each item. Consider the elimination or redefinition of items where the responses show no or very little variation; consider redefinition where

items with multiple categories are poorly scaled (most responses at one extreme and a few at the other).

(2) examine the distribution of subjects' dimension scores (whether regarded as categorical or continuous) across the complete dimension. The aim is to check that in practice the scores are distributed across the full range of the scale, as well as to gain some idea of overall shape, and the appropriate summary statistics.

(3) for multi-item dimensions examine the homogeneity of the items using measures such as inter-item correlations, the item-total correlation, split-half reliability, the Kuder-Richardson formula 20, and Cronbach's alpha coefficient, which are available in the Reliability Procedure within the SPSS package (SPSS, 1990); see Streiner and Norman (1989) for an extensive discussion of these measures. See also Bravo and Potvin (1991) for a discussion of Cronbach's alpha and its relationship with the intraclass correlation coefficient.

(4) the structure of a multi-dimensional rating scale may be examined using principal components analysis, and factor rotation with correlated as well as orthogonal factors. Such analyses require large sample sizes (several hundred), and should be confined to checking the basic structure of the overall rating scale and its components; they should not be used to produce a specific assignment of weights.

G. Testing

(1) assess the test-retest reliability of each dimension score (and perhaps each item) by repeated testing on a sample, and using limits of agreement, the coefficient of reliability (Bland and Altman 1986), or an intraclass kappa coefficient (Bloch and Kraemer 1989); again see Streiner and Norman (1989) for discussion, including determination of sample size. Test-retest reliability is a measure of the scale's stability when completed by the same subject, or observer, on two separate occasions separated by an appropriate interval of time. Here 'appropriate' implies that the interval is not so short that the subject or observer can remember the first assessment when making the second, or that the interval is so long that the second assessment is influenced by temporal changes. Possible sources for differences between test and retest assessments should be examined and eliminated.

(2) for scales which may be completed by independent observers examine the extent of inter-rater agreement (inter-observer variation). Traditionally this has been done by reporting correlation coefficients (which is incorrect), or one of the class of Cohen's kappa statistics, or an intraclass correlation coefficient. As pointed out by Brennan and Silman (1992), 'the analysis of observer variation must be a dual consideration of both agreement and bias', and consequently, attempts to summarise inter-observer variation by a single statistic may be doomed to failure. Again following the advice of Brennan and Silman (1992), it may be better to place 'more weight on the raw data than on any summary measure'; the simple plots recommended by Bland and Altman (1986) may be sufficient. An intraclass correlation coefficient should not be used without attention to the underlying statistical model (sampling theory), and interpretation of a kappa

coefficient requires some appreciation of its deficiencies (see Brennan and Silman 1992). Inter-observer variation is the focus of many current research papers and in addition to the papers already cited in this section readers are referred to Agresti (1992), Baker SG et al (1991) and Kraemer (1992). As with test-retest reliability the aim of studies of inter-observer variation is to understand its pattern and magnitude, to isolate the sources of extreme differences, and eliminate them.

(3) obtain ratings on separate, comparatively homogeneous groups of subjects, and examine the distributions of dimension scores within each; with continuous scales examine the relationship between within-group standard deviations and means by plotting both on logarithmic scales to assess the need for score transformations. If possible choose transformations which provide stable standard deviations (or variances), and approximately Normal distributions of scores within groups;

(4) when relevant assess the scale's ability to measure changes over time (Streiner and Norman (1989), chapter 11). Here we require reassurance that when the underlying state of a subject remains stable the rating scale itself stays relatively constant, while a change of state is followed by a change in rating. This is a problem of calibration which requires evaluation of the underlying state independently of the rating itself. A crude approach is to plot the scale changes against the state changes (overall and stratified by initial state), and then make a visual assessment; with ordered categorical scales cross-tabulations may be used. Extreme changes in rating scale not associated with state changes, as well as minor changes in rating but with marked change in state, require investigation. See Bohrnstedt (1983) for discussion of some more complicated procedures.

(5) assess the scale's ability to detect differences between treatments. Once all the previous steps have been completed this one will follow without further research. The properties of the scale will be understood, together with the change on the rating scale considered of importance when comparing two or more treatments. This information is sufficient to enable determination of sample size for an appropriately designed clinical trial; this sample size can then be compared with those determined when using other measures of comparative efficacy.

(6) compare parallel forms of the rating scale when these are available, and assess association with other relevant scales.

H. Packaging

(1) produce a packaged version of the scale, including a guide to its completion and use, as well as information about its properties and how it should be analyzed.

TIME DEPENDENT COVARIATES

The "survival-type" analyses described earlier can be extended within the framework of the Cox proportional hazards regression model to examine the effect of patient and disease characteristics upon subsequent risk of seizure recurrence (or any other "event of interest"). Indeed this multivariate approach was used to identify factors of prognostic importance in the AEDWS (Medical Research Council Antiepileptic Drug Withdrawal Study Group 1991), and more recently to develop a model to predict the risk of seizure recurrence under policies of continued treatment, and slow AED withdrawal. In these analyses the prognostic factors are "fixed" in that their values are determined at "base-line," that is prior to the start of follow-up, and no account is taken of later changes. However the Cox model can be extended to factors (usually called covariates) which are allowed to vary over time. Such models offer some opportunity to investigate more complex inter-relationships, for example the effects of varying AED serum concentrations on risk of seizure recurrence. So far they have not been exploited in epilepsy. Two recent examples concern surrogate markers for survival in patients with AIDS (Jacobsen et al 1991), and ipsilateral breast tumour recurrence after lumpectomy (Fisher et al 1991).

MULTISTATE MODELS

Earlier we discussed the analysis of intervals from a specified starting date to an "event of interest," such as first seizure recurrence, or a remission period of one year; the choice of one year was described as arbitrary. A characteristic of these analyses was restriction to just one single "event." beyond which the seizure or remission pattern was ignored. Since epilepsy is a recurrent condition it is natural to question what happens after an initial "event," and in particular whether its occurrence signals a change in the risk of further seizures. For example, we may wish to estimate the chances of a second year in remission after the first, or whether the risk of seizure recurrence changes (perhaps declines) following each successive year of remission. Such questions are arbitrary in that they can be framed in a multitude of ways, but all have a common framework in the definition of a number of disease states between which patients transfer during follow-up; such models underpin "event history analysis" (Clayton 1988). An example with four disease states is shown in Figure 3.

We assume that patients start from a nominated date (for example date of randomisation or date of an index seizure) in state 1, and remain there until they attain a 6 month remission period, when they transfer to state 2; subsequently they either move to state 3 (after a further 6 months in remission) or return to state 1 after seizure recurrence and perhaps begin the cycle again. The percentages of patients in each state throughout the follow-up period, as well as the transfer intensities between them and their time-dependence can be estimated and plotted.

Multistate models are extremely flexible and offer one opportunity for modelling the progression of epilepsy over time. In the example the states relate to seizure recurrence, but in principle there is no reason why they should be defined solely in these terms; they could for example relate to whether or not a patient is prescribed AED's, whether a patient is employed, psychosocial status, and so on. Such models therefore offer some hope of eventually studying and understanding the complex disease, treatment and social interactions which characterise epilepsy. Essentially they require sensible definition of a small number of states, and an adequate set of data with which to work. There is a vast

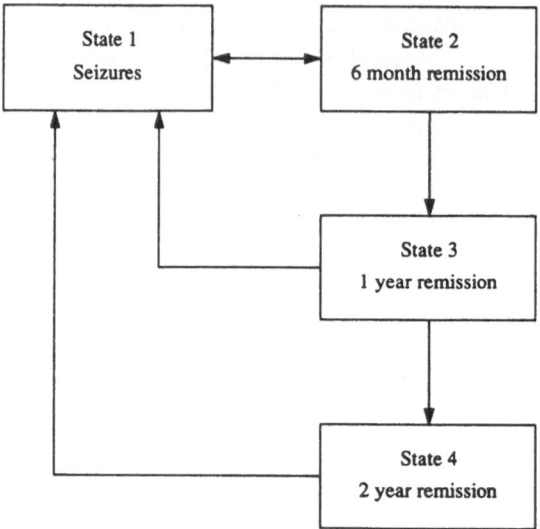

Figure 3. Multistate model for seizure recurrence.

literature of statistical theory, but at present a lack of readily implemented, user-friendly computer software. As yet these new techniques have not been used in epilepsy; an example from a study of nephropathy in diabetes is provided by Andersen (1988).

CONCLUSION

The methodology for handling the analysis of complex recurrent events, and their interactions with the broader social and psychosocial aspects of life is only now emerging from the realms of statistical theory. Hopefully its implementation in computer programs will soon enable the detailed analyses which will lead to the better understanding of epilepsy (and other recurrent disorders) for which we have waited so long. Seizure recurrence, point processes and the theory of martingales may sound a long way apart; in practice they may be of great mutual benefit.

REFERENCES

Agresti A. Categorical data analysis. New York: Wiley. 1990.

Agresti A. Modelling patterns of agreement and disagreement. Statistical Methods in Medical Research 1992:1:201–218.

Altman DG. Practical statistics for medical research. London.:Chapman and Hall. 1991.

Andersen PK. Multistate models in survival analysis: a study of nephropathy and mortality in diabetes. Statistics in Medicine 1988; 7:661–670.

Annegers JF et al. Remission of seizures and relapse in patients with epilepsy. Epilepsia 1979:20:729–737.

Baker GA et al. The development of a seizure severity scale as an outcome measure in epilepsy. Epilepsy Research 1991:8:245–251.

Baker SG et al. Using replicate observations in observer agreement studies with binary assessments. Biometrics 1991:47:1327–1338.

Bland JM and Altman DG. Statistical methods for assessing agreement between two methods of çlinical measurement. Lancet 1986:i:307–310.

Bloch DA and Kraemer HC. 22 Kappa coefficients: measures of agreement or association. Biometrics 1989:45:269–287.

Bravo G and Potvin L. Estimating the reliability of continuous measures with Cronbach's alpha or the intraclass correlation coefficient: towards the integration of two traditions. Journal of Clinical Epidemiology 1991:44:381–390.

Brennan P and Silman A. Statistical methods for assessing observer variability in clinical measures. British Medical Journal 1992:304:1491–1494.

Bohrnstedt GW. Measurement. In Rossi, PH et al. eds. Handbook of Survey Research. New York: Academic Press: 1983:69–121.

Clayton DG. The analysis of event history data: a review of progress and outstanding problems. Statistics in Medicine 1988:7:819–841.

Coatsworth JJ. Studies on the clinical efficacy of marketed antiepileptic drugs. NINDS Monograph no 12, DHEW Pub no (NIH) 73–51,1971.

Cox DR et al. Quality-of-life assessment: can we keep it simple? Journal of the Royal Statistical Society, Series A 1992:155:353–375.

Cramer JA et al. A method of quantification for the evaluation of antiepileptic drug therapy. Neurology 1983:331(suppl 1):26–37.

Duncan JS and Sander JWAS. The Chalfont seizure severity scale. Journal of Neurology, Neurosurgery and Psychiatry 1991:54:873–876.

Feinstein AR. Clinimetrics. New Haven: Yale University Press. 1987.

Fisher B et al. Significance of ipsilateral breast tumour recurrence after lumpectomy. Lancet 1991:338:327–331.

Fleiss JL. Statistical methods for rates and proportions. New York.:Wiley. 1981.

Fleiss JL. Williams JBW. Dubro AF. The logistic regression analysis of psychiatric data. Journal of Psychiatric Research 1986:20:195–209

Goodridge DMG and Shorvon SD. Epileptic seizures in a population of 6000. I.Demography, diagnosis and classification, and role of the hospital services. British Medical Journal 1983:287:641–644.

Gordon RE. An introduction to psychiatric research. Cambridge: Cambridge University Press. 1988.

Hart YM et al. National General Practice Study of Epilepsy: recurrence after a first seizure. Lancet 1990:338:1271–1274.

Hosmer DW and Lemeshow S. Applied logistic regression. New York: Wiley. 1989.

Jacobsen MA et al. Surrogate markers for survival in patients with AIDS and AIDS related complex treated with zidovudine. British Medical Journal 1991:302:73–78.

Jawad S et al. Controlled trial of Lamotrigine (Lamictal) for refractory seizures. Epilepsia 1989:30:356–363.

Jones B and Kenward MG. Design and analysis of cross-over trials. London: Chapman and Hall. 1989.

Knippenberg van FCE and de Haes JCJM. Measuring the quality of life of cancer patients: psychometric properties of instruments. Journal of Clinical Epidemiology 1988:41:1043–1053.

Kraemer HC. Measurement of reliability for categorical data in medical research. Statistical Methods in Medical Research 1992:1:183–199.

Medical Research Council Antiepileptic Drug Withdrawal Study Group. Randomised study of antiepileptic drug withdrawal in patients in remission. Lancet 1991:337:1175–1180.

Morley S and Snaith P. Principles of psychological assessment. In Freeman C and Tyrer P. eds. Research methods in psychiatry. London: Royal College of Psychiatrists. 2nd edition. 1992:135–152.

Peto R et al. Design and analysis of randomised clinical trials requiring prolonged observation of each patient: I. Introduction and design, II. Analysis and examples. British Journal of Cancer 1976:34:585–612 and 1977:35:1–39.

SPSS Base System User's Guide. SPSS Inc. 1990.

Streiner DL and Norman GR. Health measurement scales: a practical guide to their development and use. Oxford:Oxford University Press. 1989.

Taber's Cyclopedic Medical Dictionary 15th edition. Philadelphia: Davis. 1985.

Thompson CT. ed. The instruments of psychiatric research. Chichester:Wiley. 1989.

Turnbull DM et al. Which drug for the adult epileptic patient: phenytoin or valproate? British Medical Journal 1985:290:815–819.

SEIZURE FREQUENCY AS TREATMENT EFFECT PARAMETER: GENERAL CONSIDERATIONS

M.W. Lammers, M.D. and H. Meinardi, M.D., Ph.D.

Institute of Neurology
University Hospital St. Radboud
Catholic University Nijmegen
Nijmegen, The Netherlands

INTRODUCTION

As epilepsy is a paroxysmal disorder it seems self-evident that the frequency of occurrence of paroxysms is a sensible index. However, as Feinstein admonishes in his teachings on clinimetrics, the first question to be asked is for what purpose do we intend to use the index.

If we simply wish to know what chance we have in a given period to register a seizure, the bare frequency will offer an estimate. If we wish to study the influence of different conditions on the occurrence of one type of seizures in one patient, again frequency per se will suffice. If we wish to study the impact of seizures on the quality of life of the patient seizure frequency per se is no longer sufficient. If two seizure types occur in the same patient, and if these types are related (e.g., complex partial and secondarily generalized seizures), the occurrence of the one excluding the presence of the other while the seizure-type-specific seizure frequency differs, then simple counting of events per period will not be meaningful. If indexes are needed to evaluate different interventions in groups of people with epilepsy, simply referring to the seizure frequency may not be relevant. A case in point is the custom to assess the efficacy of anti-epileptic drugs by measuring percent change in seizure frequency. Such a choice implies that it should not make any difference in the efficacy of a drug whether it provides a reduction of 50% in seizure frequency in a patient suffering from 4 generalized tonic-clonic seizures a day, or in a patient who suffered from 4 generalized tonic-clonic seizures a week, or for that matter from 4 generalized tonic-clonic seizures a year. Whether the differences in inherent frequency and in therapy-resistance between different seizure-types are harmonized by assessing the changes in frequency by percentage is doubtful. When the efficacy of an

Quantitative Assessment in Epilepsy Care, Edited by H. Meinardi et al.
Plenum Press, New York, 1993

29

anti-epileptic drug is assessed by summing up the frequencies of all seizure types, several authors have applied (presumably intuitively) weighting coefficients.[1,2] The effect of clustering of seizures is more or less provided for by taking a study period of sufficient length, however, other diseases or patient related periodicities in seizure frequency are rarely ever accounted for.

A scrutiny of ten randomly selected trails of anti-epileptic drugs reveals that most authors identify in the inclusion criteria at least a demarcating lowest seizure frequency, but do not try to obtain a fairly homogeneous study group as far as seizure frequency is concerned. Many but not all mention seizure type and group participants according to the individual pattern of seizure type(s). Even those authors consider seizures regardless of type as equivalent events, and present change as percentage seizures with respect to a baseline period. Occasionally a specific seizure type is analyzed separately, however, without mentioning whether patients were included with only a single seizure type.

Change in Seizure Frequency as a Clinimetric Index

Let us examine **change in seizure frequency** with the help of the checklist which Feinstein has provided to appraise the sensibility of this index.[3]

Purpose and Framework

The index is clearly disorder specific. The function is to measure the transit between two states. The clinical justification to select seizure frequency is supported by the fact that seizures are the typical manifestations of epilepsy, however, the point of debate is whether specific seizures are the manifestations to focus on or whether the type of seizure is irrelevant for the severity of the disease process.

The applicability of seizure counts is reasonable as seizures are behavioral manifestations that can be easily detected. A cautionary remark is, however, that in case of certain seizure types the patient may not be aware that a seizure occurred. Recording of seizures in that case will depend on the presence of an observer (or in theory a registering device).

Comprehensibility

As far as comprehensibility is concerned seizure frequency is a simple concept; sometimes there are several variables included (e.g. in studying patients with a Lennox Gastaut syndrome, Illum et al.[4] distinguished Absence seizures, Tonic seizures, Myoclonic seizures and Atonic seizures). This index, contrary to the Index of Seizures[2,5] does not use weighting factors; the biological connotation is clear.

Replicability

Replicability seems guaranteed, however, in practice problems may arise if some of the patients under study have seizures that occur in series with very brief intervals. Even though such series may comprise twenty or thirty distinct seizures, many authors would consider them as a manifestation of a single epileptic event comparable with status epilepticus. Replicability may also be jeopardized if the situation of the patient changes from having an observer present or not.

Suitability of Scale

With respect to the suitability of the scale one may argue that seizure frequency is insufficiently comprehensive as no account is given of elements like seizure duration, predictability of the seizure occurrence, presence or absence of an aura. Overweg[6] mentioned that in a clinical trial of flunarizine patients were unhappy with the drug even though their seizure frequency diminished for in those seizures that persisted the aura was no longer noticeable. Seizure frequency per se fulfils the requirement of easy discrimination; percent change in seizure frequency, however, does not as was stated before.

Face Validity

The face validity of seizure frequency may be less strong as patients may differ in opinion which behavioral manifestations are part of an ictal event.

The focus of basic evidence usually is a mark made by the patient on a seizure calendar, if a phenomenon has occurred which the patient and the physician have agreed to consider a seizure. Biologic coherence of components is not an issue because the index is only comprised of one component.

With respect to personal collaboration appraisal enters the realm of compliance studies. This is a context dependent problem. In clinical trials a double-blind study format neutralizes collaboration problems in an individual scale, though an impact on group analysis remains.

Content Validity and Ease of Usage

The discussion of content validity repeats the discussion about the suitability of seizure frequency as an index. The widespread use of this index in the literature is proof of its ease of usage.

DISCUSSION

Seizure frequency can also be used in assessing the difference in seizure frequency in different types of seizures. Reynolds et al.[7] performed a study for assessing the efficacy of phenytoin as monotherapy in newly diagnosed patients with generalized tonic clonic seizures, and patients with partial seizures, both with simple and complex symptomatology. There was a marked difference in seizure frequency between the two aforementioned seizure types. Before therapy the seizure frequency for generalized tonic clonic seizures was 0.95 attacks/month compared to 8.15 attacks/month for partial seizures. After optimalisation of the phenytoin levels the frequency for generalized tonic clonic seizures was 0.01 attacks/month compared to 0.60 attacks/month for partial seizures.

In spite of the ease of usage of seizure frequency as an index, several authors felt the need to improve this index. Meinardi[1] decided to affix weighting factors to the counts of generalized tonic clonic, complex partial and absence seizures. The aim was to facilitate comparison of efficacy between patients suffering from different seizure types. The coefficients were intuitively assigned according to the difference in seizure frequency manifested by the aforementioned seizure types.

Cramer et al.[2] modified seizure counts first according to type of seizure, generalized tonic clonic seizures collected twice as many points as complex partial seizures, and the latter again collected about three times as many points as simple partial seizures. Neither Meinardi nor Cramer et al. appear to have based their scoring differences on epidemiological studies of seizure counts. Cramer et al. also modified their counts by terms that would refer to seizure severity. Seizure severity is a separate topic of discussion and will be dealt with further on. Furthermore Cramer et al. constructed a composite score, designed to reflect the total effect of seizures and toxicity of medication on the quality of life of the patient. This score is the summation of seizure frequency rating, systemic toxicity rating and a combination of neurotoxicity and behavioral toxicity ratings. So the composite score is an example of differentiation by seizure type and differential attribution of point scores. Wijsman et al.[5] validated a similar Composite Index of Impairment by testing the correlation of the independently assessed score by the investigator with the interval between clinic visits ordained by the physician in charge of the patient. Wijsman et al., however, did not compare this correlation with the correlation of either the frequency of seizures per se, or the frequency of seizures weighted according to seizure type. Smith et al.[8] constructed a patient-based severity scale to analyze the relationship between seizure severity, seizure frequency and psychological factors such as anxiety, self-esteem and locus of control. Based on the study Smith expects that seizure frequency alone may not be sensitive enough to assess the efficacy of anti-epileptic drugs. Several other others have indicated that seizure frequency alone will not be sufficient in assessing the severity of epilepsy.[9,10] Martins da Silva et al.[11] on the other hand has shown that seizure frequency is a relevant parameter if the seizure characteristics remain constant. On pursuing the introduction of clinimetrics in epilepsy care further analysis of the advantage of the possible scores is undoubtedly needed.

Acknowledgement: This work was supported by a grant of CLEO-NEF (Netherlands).

REFERENCES

1. H. Meinardi, Clinical trials of anti-epileptic drugs, *Psychiat.Neurol.Neurochir.* 74, 141, (1971).
2. J.A. Cramer, D.B. Smith, R.H. Mattson et al. A method of quantification for the evaluation of anti-epileptic drugtherapy. *Neurology* 33(suppl.): 26–37 (1983)
3. A.R. Feinstein, Clinimetrics. Yale University Press, New Haven (1987).
4. N. Illum, K. Taudorf, C. Heilmann, et.al. Intravenous immunoglobulin in a single-blind trial in children with Lennox-Gastaut syndrome,*Neuropediatrics.* 21:87 (1990).
5. D.J.P. Wijsman, Y.A. Hekster, A. Keyser et al., Clinimetrics and epilepsy care, Pharm. Weekbl. [Sc.], 13: 182, (1991).

6. J. Overweg, D. Ashton, F. de Beukelaar, et al., Add-on therapy in epilepsy with calcium entry blockers, Eur. Neurol.: 25 suppl.1:93, (1986).

7. E.H. Reynolds, S.D. Shorvon, A.W. Galbraith et al. Phenytoin monotherapy for epilepsy: a longterm prospective study, assisted by serum level monitoring, in previously untreated patients. *Epilepsia* 22: 475, (1981).

8. D.F. Smith, G.A. Baker, M. Dewey, et al., Seizure frequency, patient-perceived seizure severity and the psychosocial consequences of intractable epilepsy. *Epilepsy Res.* 9: 231, (1991).

9. J.S. Duncan, J.W.A.S. Sander, The Chalfont seizure severity scale, *J. Neurol., Neurosurg., and psychiatry* 54: 873, (1991).

10. G.A. Baker, D.F. Smith, M.Dewey et al., The development of a seizures severity scale as an outcome measure in epilepsy. *Epilepsy Res.* 8: 245, (1991).

11. A. Martins da Silva, E. Lourenço, J.M. Nunes and D. Mendonça, Seizure frequency as treatment effect parameter, this volume 35

SEIZURE FREQUENCY AS TREATMENT EFFECT PARAMETER

A. Martins da Silva, M.D., Ph.D.,[1,2] E. Lourenço, M.D.,[1]
J.M. Nunes, BsC.,[3] and D. Mendonça, Ph.D.[3]

[1]Serviço de Neurofisiologia
Hospital Geral de Santo António
[2]Unidade de Fisiologia Humana
[3]Unidade de Biometria
Instituto Ciências Biomédicas Abel Salazar
Universidade do Porto
4000 Porto, Portugal

INTRODUCTION

Efficacy measurement of epilepsy treatment is frequently overwhelmed by the multiple variables involved: interactions between antiepileptic drugs are sometimes inextricable (Gram et al., 1981); and seizure factors (pattern, severity and frequency) have different degrees of importance on patient status (neurological, psychiatric or psychological well–being) influencing epilepsy evolution. These variables are important not only for epilepsy prognosis but they also tend to operate whatever the stage of epilepsy (Shorvon, 1984). The lack of objective measures of data, the quantification of all intervening variables (from the seizures and from the patients), the side-effects of drugs, the patient–to–patient differences, the length of disease, the duration of study design and sample dimensions are supplementary difficulties in epilepsy assessment. How to manage such variables in order to establish stable and reproducible criteria to assess epilepsy evolution or how to measure the relevance of factors as indexes of the evolution of this clinical phenomena are questions to be addressed by a clinimetric approach (Feinstein, 1987). Introducing concepts of clinimetrics with parametrization of appropriate epilepsy indexes, seizure components were used to assess epilepsy evolution. Rating scales were developed in order to solve some difficulties in the assessment of antiepileptic drugs (AED) efficacy.

As reduction of seizure frequency and tabulations of the percentages of reduction of the number of seizures are only addressing to one aspect of drug efficacy, seizure severity as a function of seizure type was combined with seizure frequency and toxicity (systemic

Quantitative Assessment in Epilepsy Care, Edited by H. Meinardi et al.
Plenum Press, New York, 1993

35

and neurologic) ratings. These combined or composite scores were developed to assess the effect of seizures and the relevance of toxicity on patients quality of life (Cramer et al., 1983; Mattson et al., 1985). The sum scores of seizure factors: type and frequency rating, with systemic and neurological ratings give the total composite score. The rating scores start from zero—the ideal end point of a good epilepsy treatment. The usual outpatient population of epileptics is within the range of 0–50. Scores higher than 50 reflect the worst epilepsy cases with bad seizure control. This type of composite scales was found to be useful to test efficacy of AED treatment and seizure evolution (Cramer et al., 1983; Mattson et al., 1985; Wijsman et al., 1991).

Further developments of seizure scales have addressed objective aspects of severity (Duncan and Sander, 1991) or more subjective i.e. patient perception of seizure severity (Baker et al., 1991). By such approaches the efficacy of epilepsy treatment was determined as a result of the combination of the advantages of seizure relief or changes on severity indexes with the inconveniences of the impairments resulting from antiepileptic drugs' side-effects. These scales will be useful when applied in longitudinal studies, when the epilepsy progresses and patient rates at different moments can be compared (Duncan and Sander, 1991). They give important measures to assess severity of the individual seizure types without giving, however, the global assessment of epilepsy severity. For other authors, in clinical trials, the seizure frequency was the pertinent effect parameter (Gram et al., 1981), the primary endpoint of efficacy (Van Belle and Temkin, 1983) or the relevant factor for determination of drug description pattern (Keyser et al., 1990). These authors use seizure frequency as the traditional method of assessing response to an antiepileptic drug, in which any decrease in fit frequency was considered as a parameter of efficacy (Milligan and Richens, 1981). In specific types of epilepsy the quantification of the frequency of the epileptic phenomena, both seizures and/or EEG epileptiform events, was used as excellent parameter of seizure control as for instance in children with clinical absences and spike and wave discharges. Although the general pattern of seizure frequency is relatively stable, the consistency of day–to–day profile of EEG epileptiform events (or amount of interictal epileptiform activity) seemed more dependent on the basic rest–activity cycle rather than on the direct antiepileptic drug influence (Martins da Silva et al., 1984; Duncan, 1987). However frequency alone is insufficient as a measure or effect parameter in epilepsy treatment. In some cases a 75% reduction in seizure frequency could be a therapeutic failure if the patient would remain seizure disabled (Baker et al., 1991), requiring more knowledge of different seizure variables.

Quantitative scales are useful in long–term follow up of patients with recurrent seizures to determine the efficacy of new drugs. However, when the seizure pattern is severity stable, i.e., almost constant severity, while frequency is changing, frequency is also the relevant parameter in the assessment of epilepsy evolution. In such situations the evolution of the patient's outlook can be based on seizure frequency quantification.

Finally, in the assessment of the efficacy of an antiepileptic treatment and consequent patient epilepsy prognosis, the interindividual variables, such as the psychological consequences and/or patients quality of life, have only recently been introduced as factors on scales (Baker et al, 1991; Smith et al., 1991). Seizure frequency is an important parameter of epileptic patient quality of life (Baker et al., 1991; Smith et al., 1991) and patients well being (Taveira et al., subm.). Although inappropriately used by some authors as the sole end point of the efficacy parameter, it is the experience of many clinicians that many patients complain about seizure frequency being used as the most relevant factor of their epilepsy outcome. Taking these aspects into consideration we used seizure frequency to define epilepsy evolution in a group of chronic epileptic patients regularly followed up for more than three years. We assessed the relevance of seizure frequency in different ways: i) seizure frequency was used as sole end points to test drug efficacy; ii) seizure frequency was tested as a relevant factor for patient well-being; iii) seizure frequency was tested as a factor to assess epilepsy evolution.

METHODS AND RESULTS

Seizure Frequency as Endpoint of AED Treatment

The relevance of seizure frequency as primary end point was studied in a group of seven school children with absences. Patients were selected at the first consultation in the

Table 1. Computer analysis of spike and wave discharges. Patients 1 to 7 were reported before and after treatment with ESM = ethosuximide and VPA = valproic acid.

Pat. N.	N. of Discharges			Duration		Spike		Slow Wave		Rep.
	< 3 (sec)	3–10 (sec)	> 10 (sec)	Total (sec)	Mean (sec)	Amp (μv)	Half dur.	Amp (μv)	Half dur.	Period (sec)
1	18	7	1	91.8	8.2	193	.053	272	.15	.36
ESM	**14**	**3**	**0**	**32.2**	**5.1***	**163**	**.065***	**124****	**.13****	**.32***
2	39	17	1	165.1	6.1	157	.055	228	.16	.39
VPA	**26**	**6**	**0**	**57.1**	**4.2**	**157**	**.046***	**180**	**.13****	**.34****
3	39	5	6	163.4	10.3	226	.047	309	.17	.36
VPA	**1**	**0**	**5**	**85.6**	**15.9****	**180**	**.048**	**207****	**.17**	**.36**
4	34	2	4	120.4	13.4	197	.055	428	.19	.39
VPA	**32**	**12**	**4**	**151.8**	**7.1****	**131****	**.049**	**174****	**.14****	**.34****
5	73	5	0	98.1	4.1	170	.052	170	.14	.36
ESM	**0**	**0**	**0**							
6	6	9	0	55.8	4.6	196	.057	281	.17	.38
ESM	**0**	**0**	**0**							
7	5	3	7	192.1	17.7	203	.049	194	.14	.32
ESM	**0**	**0**	**0**							

Bold figures: parameters after medication. Significance level: *p < 0.05, **p < 0.01 (F test).
Rep. = repetition period.

outpatient clinic. Immediately after, they have been submitted to an EEG and videore-cording during six hours to assess the epilepsy diagnosis. The number and characteristics of seizures and discharges were recorded just before starting treatment. EEG signal was also recorded on analog tape and digitized. Computer detection and analysis of spike and wave discharges (duration of events, amplitude and repetition period) were performed on line (Tomé et al., 1985). The patients under treatment (VPA or ESM) were monitored six months later under the same conditions.

As shown in table 1 the seizures frequency and spike and wave discharges de-creased, being suppressed in 3 patients. Significant changes on temporal characteris-tics of spike and wave events were found: amplitude and duration values of each spike and/or slow wave parameters, as well as their repetition periods, have been reduced after treatment. Frequency and duration of seizures are, in such cases, treatment effect parameters.

Seizure Frequency as Relevant Factor for Patient Well-being

In a group of 80 adult epileptic patients, with recurrent seizures we tested the rele-vance of seizure frequency on patients well-being. Self–esteem was assessed by means of a Portuguese Adapted Version of the Adult Self Perception Profile–ASPP (Messer and Harter, 1986). Patients had chronic recurrent seizures (Generalized TC; Partial: S or C; Myoclonic; or multiple types) and no other illness or handicap and were able to lead a regular social, professional or family life. In this group of patients, the presence of fits was significantly associated with decrease in sociability / intimate relationship and humour. Using analysis of variance methods it was shown that the mean score in this domain was significantly lower for patients with seizures than for those without seizures. Epileptic patients who have had seizures during the year before evaluation felt less adequate and competent in social situations than those whose seizures were well con-trolled (Taveira et al., in press).

Seizure Frequency as a Factor to Assess Epilepsy Evolution

From the population of epileptic outpatients with recurrent but stable types of sei-zures, a group of 9 was retrospectively analyzed. Those patients were selected by review-ing their medical records, and have been chosen from those who have been followed up for a period of more than three years. The influence of seizure frequency on epilepsy evolution was studied. Patients had a well defined history of seizures always of the same characteristics, recurring frequently in spite of good response of seizure severity to antiepileptic treatment. All but two had complex partial seizures. The remainder had simple partial seizures. All of them had, in the past, rare generalized tonic clonic seizures. The patients complained of changing levels of seizure disability in spite of the stabilized seizure severity. Only patients with reliable and consistent data remained on the study.

The information on the relevance of seizure severity was taken from the medical records, from patient diaries and family witness reports. The patients and their families registered the number and the type of seizures noting if any change had occurred. Patients were examined every three months. The plots of seizure frequency showed marked fluctuations in spite of the stability of the remaining seizure characteristics. In all but the last examination the analysis was done retrospectively. In the last examination the severity score was established by applying the Chalfont scale. The Chalfont scale was selected because it is considered to be an adequate scale for longitudinal studies of seizure severity (Duncan and Sander, 1991). If the information from the medical record describing seizure severity characteristics remained stable during the last consultations and the stability was confirmed by patient and family information we took this severity value and applied it retrospectively, only adapting the scores to the minor changes as they were reported. Such use of scales although controversial could be effective to control the stability of one variable—seizure severity—allowing an easier analysis of seizure frequency.

Plots of the number of seizures that had occurred in the previous 6 month periods, showed marked fluctuations giving rise to difficulties on the understanding of the impact of frequency changes (Fig. 1). In these plots the scores of the patient when he is better tend to be zero. In order to minimize the non-specificity of plots fluctuation we combined frequency with stable seizure severity scores. The simple multiplication of the values of the frequency by the severity score F × S (where F is the frequency and S is the Chalfont Score) or F × S/10 (just to provide a better graphic display as shown in figure 1) do not improve the analysis.

It was evident that the importance of seizure frequency reduction depends on the baseline. For example, the relevance of a 50% decrease from 400 to 200 seizures can, for the patient's well-being, be less representative than the change from 10 to 5 or from 6 to 3. This demands for a different analysis of the counting process. Then, a logarithmic transformation was applied in order to smooth the influence of the high number of seizures and a new composite score was calculated as **Int (S × Ln (1 + F))**. With such approach an Epilepsy Severity Score (ESS) was calculated for each one of the patients. As shown in Fig. 2 the relevance of seizure frequency is now balanced with ESS values giving a better indication of the influence of the introduction of new treatment (Clobazam) on outcome. The loss of effect of Clobazam on seizure frequency after 18 months is also seen.

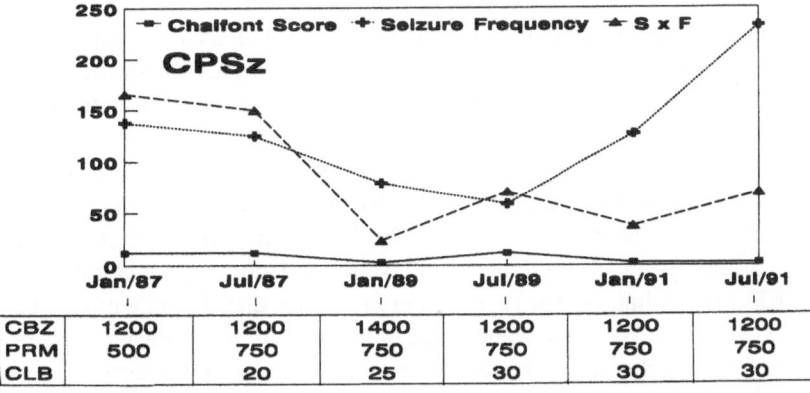

Figure 1. Plots of seizure frequency and S × F/10 showing marked fluctuations.

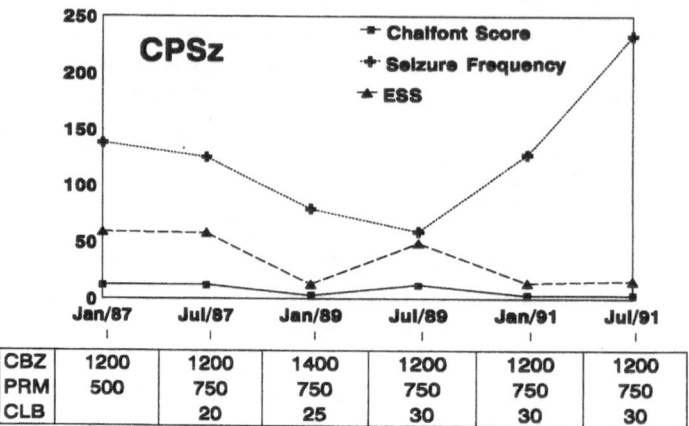

Figure 2. Plots of Chalfont scores and seizure frequency as in Figure 1 and the values of the logarithmic transformation.

This figure 2 shows that neither the single frequency analysis nor the single seizure severity analysis provides complete information on epilepsy evolution. The patient appeared to be worse at the last consultation than at the previous one. Looking at the simple plot of seizure frequency the patient had a higher number of seizures in the last six-month interval, all of them of the same severity. The clinical status was reported by the patient, family and clinicians to be worse in July 91 than in January 91, however to be considerably better than in July 89. A more appropriate picture of this epilepsy evolution was expressed by the ESS values which showed a higher value on the last consultation than in the previous one, but the value on the last consultation was much lower than that presented in July 89.

DISCUSSION

The studies we carried out in these different populations offer some points for a generalized discussion on epilepsy quantification. The examples we showed identified the importance of seizure frequency as a relevant parameter on epilepsy outcome. However, discussions about seizure frequency are often concerned solely with the counting of the number of events. Considered by itself, seizure frequency is not adequate to define epilepsy evolution apart from the study of absences in children. As we showed the evolution of the absences in children could be better studied by applying methods of quantification of temporal characteristics of events and combining counting of clinical events with EEG recording. In that case we demonstrated that the patient was better when he had fewer seizures. We also demonstrated that the time characteristics of seizures and/or epileptiform discharges were modified as a function of medication. The need to introduce different approaches or models to analyze seizure frequency was already stressed by others. Some authors got more information about seizure frequency by applying different mathematical approaches. Kogeorgos et al., 1981 applied the Cusum techniques. Based on the patient's detailed seizure registration, the mean time between attacks is calculated during a certain period. This mean is subtracted from each of the subsequent time intervals between seizures and a plot is drawn. The Cusum plot may reveal changes in seizure frequency and drug influences that might not be so obvious on a straight plot.

These approaches and those used by ourselves for the analysis of the first group of patients introduces several questions: To validate the relevance of seizure frequency on the study of epilepsy evolution what aspects of seizure frequency need to be analyzed as treatment effect parameters? Are we using the correct approach or model of analysis, to gauge the effect of seizure frequency?

In the second group of patients the influence of seizure frequency on the patient's well-being was documented. The questions we tried to answer addressed the relevance of seizure frequency on the patients' well-being and epilepsy evolution. Do the total number of seizures relate to the patient's well-being? Is the patient's perception of seizure frequency a determinant for this outcome? Is the individual relevance of such parameters objectively identified and quantified?

In the last group studied, the relevance of seizure frequency as treatment effect parameter is documented in longitudinal studies by providing evidence of the overall patient perception of the relevance of this parameter on the evolution of his disease. Although our method to "stabilize" severity scores was somewhat artificial (because we applied the scale retrospectively in all but the last examination, when the score was calculated based on a direct patient interview), as the information from patients, family and doctors agreed, we considered that the variable "severity" was controlled during the whole period. In such group of patients the small changes of seizure frequency were relevant for the outcome. Patients perceived them as changes inducing disability. This illustrates the advantages of the use of combined information as we tried with the ESS to assess epilepsy evolution and drug efficacy. Such procedure will be continued in this group of patients in a prospective way, in order to test the stability of the scores.

The data we reported using three different approaches demonstrated the relevance of seizure frequency for the study of epilepsy evolution and for the assessment of efficacy of any treatment. Development of seizure scales is different from development of epilepsy evolution scales. An Epilepsy Evolution Scale or Scales should be developed for use different from the Apgar or Glasgow Coma Scales. It should be different because unlike the expected alterations in status of babies or trauma patients (the first minutes of life of the newborn or the duration of the coma), epilepsy is a chronic disease with recurrent events in an individual, subject to different external factors. Such a scale would also differ from the traditional objective use of exclusively the seizure counts. Thus, a scale of epilepsy evolution is needed in which the patient's perception of different seizure characteristics, such as frequency, severity and predictability, as well as other relevant factors for patient's well-being might be included. It is also necessary to take into account social, professional, educational and cultural factors, all of which influence epileptic patient outcome.

REFERENCES

Baker GA, Smith DF, Dewey M, Morrow J, Crawford PM, Chadwick DW. The development of a seizure severity scale as an outcome measure in epilepsy. *Epilepsy Res.* 1991; 8:245–251.

Cramer JA, Smith DB, Mattson RH, Delgado-Escueta AV, Collins JF, Browne TR, Crill WE, Homan RW, Maysersdorf A, McCutchen CB, McNamara JO, Rosenthal NP, Treiman DM, Wilder BJ, Williamson PD. A method of quantification for the evaluation of antiepileptic drug therapy. *Neurology* 1983; 33 (Suppl):26–37.

Duncan JS. Antiepileptic drugs and the electroencephalogram. *Epilepsia* 1987; 28(3):259–266.

Duncan JS, Sander JWAS. The Chalfont seizure severity scale. *J Neurol Neurosurg Psychiatry* 1991; 54:873–875.

Feinstein AR, *Clinimetrics*. New Haven, CT. Yale University Press, 1987.

Gram L, Bentsen KD, Parnas J, Flachs H. Clinical trials in epilepsy: methods and results. In: Dam M, Gram L, Penry JK, eds. *Advances in Epileptology: the XIIth Epilepsy International symposium*. New York: Raven Press, 1981:105–112.

Kogeorgos JK, Evans S, Scott D. Methods of quantifications applicable to the assessment of progress and prognosis in epilepsy. In: British Epilepsy Association, edt. *Perspectives in Epilepsy 80–81*. Wokingham, Berkshire. 1981: 71–77.

Keyser A, Hekster Y, Schaap M, Termond E. Antiepileptic drug therapy in outpatients. *J Pharmacoepidemiol* 1990; 1(1):35–47.

Martins da Silva A, Aarts JHP, Binnie CD, Laxminarayan R, Lopes da Silva FH, Meijer JWA, Nagelkerke NJD. The circadian distribution of interictal epileptiform EEG activity. *Electroenceph clin Neurophysiol* 1983; 58(1):1–13.

Mattson RH, Cramer JA, Colins JF, Smith DB, Delgado-Escueta AV, Browne TR, Williamson PD, Treiman DM, McNamara JO, McCuttchen CB, Homan RW, Crill WE, Lubozynski MF, Rosenthal NP, Mayersdorf A. Comparison of carbamazepine, phenobarbital, phenytoin and primidone in partial and secondarily generalized tonic-clonic seizures. *N Engl J Med* 1985; 313(3):145–151.

Milligan N, Richens A. Methods of assessment of antiepileptic drugs. *Br J Clin Pharmac* 1981; 11: 443–456.

Shorvon SD. The temporal aspects of prognosis in epilepsy. *J Neurol Neurosurg Psychiat* 1984; 47: 1157–1165.

Smith DF, Baker GA, Dewey M, Jacoby A, Chadwick DW. Seizure frequency, patient-perceived seizure severity and the psychosocial consequences of intractable epilepsy. *Epilepsy Res* 1991; 9:231–241.

Taveira MC, Martins da Silva A, Mena Matos P, Borges I and Canijo M, Mendonça D. Self-esteem and Epilepsy: A comparative study in a Portuguese Population *Bolet. Epileps.* 1993 (in press).

Tomé AM, Principe JC, Martins da Silva A. Micro analysis of spike and wave bursts in childrens' EEG. *Electroenceph clin Neurophysiol* 1985; 61(3):S 113.

van Belle G, Temkin N. Design strategies in the clinical evaluation of new antiepileptic drugs. In: Pedley TA, Meldrum BS, eds. *Recent Advances in Epilepsy: Vol I*. London: Churchill Livingstone, 1983: 93–111.

Wijsman DJP, Hekster YA, Keyser A, Renier WO, Meinardi H. Clinimetric and epilepsy care. *Pharm Weekbl [Sci]* 1991; 13(4):182–188.

SEIZURE FREQUENCY AS TREATMENT EFFECT PARAMETER IN EPILEPTIC PATIENTS: A CRITICAL APPRAISAL OF THE CLINIMETRIC APPROACH

A. Keyser, M.D., Ph.D.

Institute of Neurology
University Hospital St. Radboud
Catholic University, Nijmegen
Nijmegen, The Netherlands

INTRODUCTION

In the proposed "Guidelines for clinical evaluation of antiepileptic drugs" from the Commission on Antiepileptic Drugs of the International League Against Epilepsy (1987) "Seizure frequency" is one of the evaluation parameters from late phase I studies onwards. In phase II studies other seizure related parameters are added such as length of seizure-free intervals, seizure duration and seizure pattern.

From Alvan Feinstein we learned that "clinimetric indexes are arbitrary ratings for the diverse phenomena of clinical care that are observed subjectively and that cannot be expressed in dimensional numbers" (Feinstein, 1987). Outcome measurement in patients with intractable epilepsy is a multifaceted enterprise and includes, in addition to seizure frequency, also assessment of the patient's subjective experience, of the psychosocial consequences of seizure activity and of the somatic damage brought about by the seizures.

Such a comprehensive clinical judgement on the epileptic patient may be translated into clinimetric indices. These indices are composed from both data that can be expressed in dimensional numbers and data that fall into the realm of subjective experience and cannot be expressed in dimensional numbers. The design of rating scales to assess the activity of an epileptic disorder aims at the conversion of the analogous data of the complex clinician's subjective judgement on a particular patient to the digital outcome of a more objective numerical rating assessment that is depending less on personal impressions. In this process a number of ingredients of clinical judgement are isolated because they possess the merit of being easily quantifiable and then these ingredients are com-

Quantitative Assessment in Epilepsy Care, Edited by H. Meinardi et al.
Plenum Press, New York, 1993

43

posed once again, in order to obtain a final outcome index. Seizure frequency ratings are part of this process of clinical assessment. This seemingly simple rating may be beset with a number of flaws that will be discussed here.

DATA COLLECTION

Seizure frequency is a parameter that can be obtained most readily and that at a first glance seems to correlate inversely with the success of therapy. The counting of seizures has to be done by the patient himself or by his relatives who should keep a seizure record book for this purpose. Here a flaw may be introduced because in some types of seizure the patient himself may not be aware of himself having a seizure, or the seizure may go unnoticed by his close relatives. In complex partial seizures a gradient may exist in behavioral modalities from normal variability of emotional behaviour towards frank pathological misdemeanour as a consequence of a temporal epileptic fit, the patient himself having limited awareness of being subject to a seizure within the borderline zone between the two. Also in some types of primary generalized seizures (e.g., absence, myoclonic seizures) seizure frequency reporting will be unreliable, therefore limiting the practicability of relying on the data provided by the patient himself. Therefore in these types of seizure, data collection for seizure frequency rating may become a problem.

SEIZURE FREQUENCY ASSESSMENT

From the contributions on seizure frequency earlier in this volume we should recall that seizure frequency is scored along a time axis and is expressed as the number of seizures per time unit. The interval between individual seizures may show regularity or may vary, the extreme of this irregularity resulting in the occurrence of seizure clustering. This aspect of seizure activity is not accounted for in mere seizure frequency ratings. This distribution of seizures along the time axis may change under the influence of therapy. This change of seizure frequency as related to the base line assessment contributes to clinical judgement on how successful therapy is and may be considered a cornerstone of any assessment of disease activity in epileptic patients.

Objective as this numerical data of seizure frequency may seem, several qualifications of seizure frequency introduce subjective experiential aspects. A change of seizure frequency in a patient of one seizure per six months period will affect this patient differently according to whether he usually suffers frequent seizures (say four seizures a month) or whether he has two seizures a year. This numerical value of change, therefore, always should be related to the basic or background frequency from which the study starts. A proportional change of a similar degree will not be experienced in every patient in the same way. A 100% increase of seizure frequency in the patient with two seizures a year has a different impact when compared to a 100% increase of seizure frequency in the patient with four seizures a month.

The regularity of seizure incidence in a patient also contributes to the burden of his disease. Clustering of seizures with large seizure free periods diminishes the social handicap of the patient. Thus, the pattern of seizures is an important item determining the impact of the epilepsy on the patient's functioning. So does seizure duration and the time needed by the patient to recover from the transient functional disturbance caused by a single seizure.

All these aspects of epileptic seizures are not accounted for when seizure frequency is considered as the sole criterion of disease activity. Seizure frequency ratings as the only parameter of disease control in epileptic patients is the least problematic in individual patient care. Here a N = 1 study is realized with an intensive design where the patient himself acts as his own control and if the rating is performed by an experienced clinician a good intra-rater reliability is obtained.

When comparing groups of patients with the same type of seizures, the use of seizure frequency ratings as a parameter of disease activity is accompanied by a number of biases such as the possibility of clustering and the relative difference of baseline values in individual patients that are not accounted for in a mere seizure frequency rating. Only patients with similar baseline values should be compared without additional corrections. But even under these strict conditions clinically important aspects of seizure activity will be lost if seizure frequency is the only parameter to be relied upon (Wijsman et al. 1991).

In addition to seizure frequency, antiepileptic treatment may also influence the spread of epileptic activity within the central nervous system. An isolated simple partial seizure is less disturbing for the patient than a complex partial seizure that may less easily be masked for his social environment and may infer considerably higher risks for physical harm. A secondarily generalized tonic-clonic seizure is an even more shattering experience, that often is followed by a period of slow recovery towards the patient's normal condition, causing functional impairment of considerable duration. Thus, if antiepileptic drug treatment limits the spread of epileptic activity and prevents the generation of the generalized tonic-clonic seizures previously present, while permitting a simple or complex partial seizure to occur, this antiepileptic drug effect is beneficial to the patient to a high degree although the number of seizures may not be diminished. Therefore, when accounting only for seizure frequency without attention for the characteristics of the seizure, important therapeutic achievements of antiepileptic drug therapy will be missed in the evaluation of patient outcome studies.

The comparison of efficacy of antiepileptic treatment in patients with different seizure types by means of seizure frequency rating scales only is not feasible. Seizures of various categories are so different as to function impairment caused by their occurrence that comparing antiepileptic drug efficacy in patients with different seizure types solely on the grounds of seizure number would introduce an enormous bias.

SEIZURE FREQUENCY VERSUS SEIZURE SEVERITY

The characteristics of a seizure may be modified by antiepileptic drug treatment, thus ameliorating the patients psychosocial adjustment and self experienced quality of life although seizure frequency may remain exactly the same. Assessment of the patient employing seizure frequency as the sole parameter, therefore, may fail to detect a substantial improvement of the patient's situation. Seizure severity should be included in the patient's assessment. This seizure severity, however, may be considered from a variety of view points depending on whether the subjective experience of the individual patient, the consequences for psychosocial and professional functioning or the medical risks are chosen, all factors contributing to the eventual outcome of the patient.

Cramer et al.(1983) from a survey of the literature from a period of over 30 years concluded that measuring of antiepileptic drug efficacy usually was either by reduction of the number of seizures or by the percentage of patients experiencing seizure frequency reduction. Often seizures type was ill defined and various different types of seizure in one patient were simply added together to obtain the seizure frequency score. They developed a seizure frequency rating scale for three well defined types of seizure and in addition to the seizure frequency as reported, they awarded a score to the presence of one or more seizures. In this seizure frequency rating scale, the seizure type determined the value of the awarded score with such weighting that the clinically unacceptable situation in every seizure type was reached when a score of 50 was obtained. The presence of factors modulating the impact of the seizure on the patient's functioning were accounted for thus reducing the scores obtained by mere frequency. The addition of these modulating factors essentially converts this seizure frequency rating scale into a seizure severity rating scale.

Baker et al. (1991) and Smith et al. (1991) recognized that seizure frequency is not sufficient as the only parameter to measure efficacy of antiepileptic treatment. They therefore developed a seizure severity scale and explored a possible relationship between seizure frequency, seizure severity and the psychosocial functional impairment in epileptic patients. An important finding was the fact that seizure frequency did not contribute to the variance of a large number of psychosocial consequences of having epilepsy, while seizure severity correlated significantly with a number of these factors.

Duncan and Sander (1991) constructed a seizure severity scale that could be operated independent from seizure frequency, and that has features from both a patient based and a physician based scale and is easily applied. The employment of these types of seizure severity scales opens the way for the study of the respective contributions of seizure frequency and seizure severity to functional impairment suffered by epileptic patients.

CONCLUSION

Seizure frequency and seizure severity are independent factors that should be considered when determining the burden of functional impairment the patient is suffering from his epileptic seizures, and when evaluating antiepileptic drug efficacy. This total burden can be expressed as consisting of a certain number of seizures of particular type modified by the qualitative characteristics of these seizures. As this quality of seizures is a matter of subjective judgement from both the viewpoint of the patient and of the physician, in a multicenter study on larger groups of patients, consensus is needed upon these matters before rating scales can be constructed or employed.

Acknowledgement: This work was supported by a grant of CLEO-NEF (Netherlands).

REFERENCES

Baker, G.A., Smith, D.F., Dewey, M. et al.: The development of a seizure severity scale as an outcome measure in epilepsy. Epilepsy Res. 1991:8:245–51.

Commission on Antiepileptic drugs. International League Against Epilepsy. Guidelines for Clinical Evaluation of Antiepileptic Drugs. August 1987 Revision.

Cramer, J.A., Smith, D.B., Mattson, R.H. et al.: A method of quantification for the evaluation of antiepileptic drug therapy. Neurology 1983, 33.Suppl.1:26–37.

Duncan, J.S., Sander, J.W.A.S.: The Chalfont Seizure Severity Scale. J. Neurol., Neurosurg. and Psych.: 1991:54:873–6.

Feinstein, A.R.: Clinimetrics. New Haven and London, Yale University Press 1987.

Smith, D.F., Baker, G.A., Dewey, M. et al.: Seizure frequency, patient perceived seizure severity and the psychosocial consequences of intractable epilepsy. Epilepsy Res. 1991:9:231–41.

Wijsman, D.J.P., Hekster, Y.A., Keyser, A. et al.: Clinimetrics and epilepsy care. Pharmaceutisch Weekbl. Sc. Ed.: 1991:13:182–8.

SEIZURE SEVERITY AS TREATMENT EFFECT PARAMETER

César Viteri, M.D. and José Manuel Martínez-Lage, M.D.

Departamento de Neurología
Unidad de Epilepsias
Clínica Universitaria
Universidad de Navarra
Apartado 192
31080 Pamplona, Spain

INTRODUCTION

According to the Dictionary of Epilepsies of the World Health Organization (Gastaut, 1973), epilepsy is a chronic brain disorder of various aetiologies characterized by recurrent seizures due to excessive discharge of cerebral neurones. Single or occasional epileptic seizures as well as those provoked during an acute illness should not be classified as epilepsy. The two cardinal elements of this definition are the epileptic nature of the paroxysmal event and its repetition through time.

Epilepsy is one of the most common chronic neurologic disorders. The outcome of any epileptic patient depends on the type of epileptic syndrome, the response to treatment and the interaction of the neurologic disease with general health and quality of life. For most patients, treatment of epilepsy at present means pharmacological control of seizures. Only a reduced number of them can benefit of new alternatives of treatment such as surgical excision of the epileptogenic focus.

The efficacy of antiepileptic drug treatment is usually measured by the effectiveness of antiepileptic drugs (AEDs) in suppressing seizures. The ideal antiepileptic drug is one which fully controls symptoms without side effects, but this is seldom achieved and in most patients outcome stands on a balance between control of symptoms and side-effects.

Although the overall prognosis of epilepsies is good (Annegers et al, 1979; Goodridge and Shorvon, 1983; Elwes et al, 1984; Oller-Daurella and Oller Ferrer-Vidal, 1985), treatment with antiepileptic drugs is unsuccessful in 20–25% of patients (Reynolds, 1986; Porter, 1988). These patients respond poorly or are refractory to all AEDs and develop distressing forms of chronic intractable epilepsy with uncontrolled seizures.

Quantitative Assessment in Epilepsy Care, Edited by H. Meinardi et al.
Plenum Press, New York, 1993

In most instances, particularly for investigational purposes, intractability has been defined exclusively by the repetition of seizures. Intractability is obviously related to the persistence of seizures, but it is evident that the number of seizures is not the only factor involved in prognosis. Severity of symptoms may become more important than frequency and in some syndromes it constitutes the main prognostic issue. Daily pycnoleptic absences or simple partial somatosensory seizures can hardly be considered as severe as less frequent tonic-clonic or atonic seizures.

All available AEDs are associated with side effects (Oxley et al, 1983; Hirtz and Nelson, 1985; Porter, 1986). It may be expected to have to discontinue or change antiepileptic therapy in up to 30% of patients, and virtually all will have some impairment of function (Hauser, 1986). The group of patients with medically intractable epilepsy is particularly at risk of the two most important consequences of persistence of seizures: toxicity of treatment and bad social adjustment.

THE CLINICAL MANAGEMENT OF EPILEPSY

In clinical practice it is well established that phenomenological description of seizures and their patterns of appearance should be comprehensively described in order to arrive to the right syndromic diagnosis and hence to the selection of the appropriate treatment. Besides reviewing of aetiology, assessment of treatment efficacy through time by means of periodic evaluation of control of seizures, side effects and quality of life is the main concern of the physician through the rest of the disease.

The whole clinical assessment of epilepsy is oriented by the clinical method to an objective evaluation and measure of disease related phenomena. Nevertheless, regarding evaluation of therapeutics and prognosis there has been traditionally a lack of objective means to assess other characteristics of seizures than frequency. It is noteworthy that seizure severity has been neglected as a clinical parameter for the classification of epilepsies or as a measure of treatment efficacy. Textbooks of clinical neurology (Adams and Victor, 1989; Rowland, 1989) and even those more comprehensive on epilepsy (Porter, 1984; Porter and Morselli, 1985; Hopkins, 1987; Dam and Gram, 1991) do not deal specifically with the evaluation of seizure severity.

It is generally accepted that the success of treatment can be equated to the absolute control of seizures with absent or minimal side effects, letting the patient lead a normal life. Treatment effects other than reduction of seizures frequency, such as modifications of the characteristics of seizures or their impact on health and social adjustment are considered so difficult to assess accurately and objectively that these are considered only collaterally, neglected or even criticized (Van Belle and Temkin, 1981).

Frequency Assessment

The frequency, number per unit of time, and the pattern of repetition over time, (i.e., clustering), are the most easily measurable characteristics of epileptic seizures. In most instances patients are encouraged to keep a record of the occurrence of seizures. Frequency of seizures as the only method of assessment of treatment efficacy is clearly inadequate since it ignores the weight of epilepsy as a personal, family and social experience. As noted before, frequent mild seizures that do not interfere with normal performance in daily living are less troublesome than a few unpredictable seizures with loss of consciousness and falling. Other alternatives of evaluation certainly need to be considered. There is agreement in that a patient based assessment of seizure severity as part of an overall quality of life measure would be the most appropriate (Baker et al, 1991; Duncan and Sander, 1991; Wijsman, 1991).

Severity Assessment

Severity of seizures has a different meaning for patients and doctors. Patients estimate not only intensity or duration of symptoms; impact of sudden, unexpected epileptic seizures on daily activities can outweigh their clinical severity, i.e., partial complex seizures may be more handicapping for an active businessman than for an unemployed patient.

There are several issues that complicate severity assessment from both patients and doctors points of view: for neurologists, severity of seizures is mainly related to their clinical and electrophysiological manifestations, and a number of clinical markers can be drawn from the clinical characteristics of seizures reflected in the classification of ILAE (Commission on Classification and Terminology of the ILAE, 1981). Severity can be gauged objectively through changes in level of consciousness, evolution to generalization with tonic-clonic convulsions or muscular tone changes leading to postural tone loss and falls, length of the ictal event and of the postictal confusion. The most severe being generalized seizures implying loss of consciousness, convulsions and sudden changes in muscular tone leading to unpreventable falls. Partial complex seizures may also be accompanied by postural tone modifications and followed by a period of confusion of variable length.

Patients, on the other hand, include in their estimation of the severity of seizures those clinical aspects they are aware of, as well as others related to their impact on quality of life. For most patients, prolonged loss of consciousness with slow postictal recovery and unpreventable falls constitute the highest degree of severity due to the risk of injuries and significant interference with labour and social activities. Seizures can disrupt performance at work, limit or impede sports practice, preclude driving motor vehicles, impair access to work or limit promotion, and many other matters.

Although in routine clinical practice patients with uncontrolled seizures are encouraged to keep a record of events, these are usually limited to the evaluation of the types and frequency of seizures. Patients tend to develop an intuitive scale to assess severity. Some of the terms often used, such as mild, moderate or severe, are ambiguous and almost impossible to translate into quantitative terms. Clinical markers of severity may be hidden by social considerations. For many patients loss of consciousness is the initial symptom so they are not aware of the subsequent details of their seizures. Witnesses or relatives often can not offer more detailed observations.

SEIZURE SEVERITY AS ASSESSMENT OF TREATMENT EFFICACY

The development of the International Classifications of Seizures (Commission on Classification and Terminology of the ILAE, 1981) and of Epilepsies and Epileptic Syndromes (Commission on Classification and Terminology of the ILAE, 1989) undoubtedly has improved diagnostic accuracy and therapeutic decisions. Nevertheless, the severity of epileptic seizures as a measure of treatment efficacy and its impact on quality of life has been traditionally neglected or evaluated only in a vague manner. Overlook of these important aspects has been due to the lack of systems for their evaluation in routine clinical practice.

The need for accurate assessment of the efficacy and adverse effects of already introduced and new antiepileptic drugs under clinical investigation has encouraged the development of comprehensive scales for assessment of treatment efficacy. In the last few years, some patient based seizure severity scales have been developed. The first (Cramer et al, 1983) was designed exclusively for assessment of new antiepileptic drugs, but subsequent scales (Baker et al, 1991; Duncan and Sander, 1991; Wijsman, 1991) have been conceived as instruments useful for comprehensive evaluation of the impact of epilepsy in daily practice.

Assessment of seizures severity is only part of the thorough evaluation that allows to set up prognosis and to measure the success of treatment. Quantitative scales should cover all major characteristics that contribute to outcome: seizure frequency, side effects and toxicity of drugs, and social consequences of disease. Validity of this approach has been demonstrated recently (Smith et al, 1991).

The development of severity assessment scales pose several problems that need accurate and clear answers in order to design instruments that really measure what we intend them to do:

(1) The purpose of the scale. Scales for clinical application may differ widely from investigational ones. Clinical oriented scales should allow a comprehensive evaluation of therapeutic and social aspects, i.e., efficacy of treatment and quality of life. Investigational scales may be more exhaustive but focused on more limited aspects of disease, i.e., efficacy and side effects of novel AEDs.

(2) Who is going to apply the scale? The level of training of people working at highly specialized facilities and the time available allow them the use of very detailed questionnaires. On the other hand, general neurologists and general practitioners attend to a larger number of patients and the time they have is limited. Scales must be easy to apply in a few minutes while maintaining their power as measure instruments. The observations and opinions of the patient are of maximal relevance; scales that collect this information must be fitted to cultural, social and any other peculiarities. This is a big obstacle to the development of scales of widespread application.

Clinical training and practice are oriented to the evaluation of diseases as quantifiable phenomena. Signs are objective, measurable facts, easier to grasp than more elusive symptoms. In order to avoid an oversimplification of the assessment of epilepsy and to transform it in a meaningless number, index or category, it is necessary to train all people involved in health care to consider epilepsy in a different way: it should not be seen as an intermittent disease, on the contrary, it is a disease whose consequences are permanent and alter almost every aspect of patients life.

Use of scales routinely in clinical practice should be encouraged. They reflect more accurately the real efficacy of treatment on seizures and the changes, improvement or deterioration, that patients perceive on daily living. Severity scales should be patient based since they measure a subjective experience. The advantages of using quantitative data are evident: they allow better and more accurate assessment in individual cases and comparison of data in research. Scales may be used for cross-sectional and longitudinal studies, and its wide use would also facilitate accurate communication between professionals.

REFERENCES

Adams R.D., and Victor M., 1989, "Principles of Neurology," fourth edition, McGraw- Hill, New York.

Annegers J.F., Hauser W.A., and Elbeback L.R., 1979, Remission of seizures and relapse in patients with epilepsy, *Epilepsia.* 20:729.

Baker G.A., Smith D.F., Dewey M., et al., 1991, The development of a seizure severity scale as an outcome measure in epilepsy, *Epilepsy Res.* 8:245.

Commission on Classification and Terminology of the ILAE., 1981, Proposal for revised clinical and electroencephalographic classification of epileptic seizures, *Epilepsia.* 22:489.

Commission on Classification and Terminology of the ILAE., 1989, Proposal for revised classification of epilepsies and epileptic syndromes, *Epilepsia.* 30:389.

Cramer J.A., Smith D.B., Mattson R.H., et al., 1983, A method of quantification for the evaluation of antiepileptic drug therapy, *Neurology.* 33(Supp 1):26.

Dam M., and Gram L., eds., 1991, "Comprehensive Epileptology," Raven Press, New York.

Duncan J.S., and Sander W.A.S., 1991, The Chalfont seizure severity scale, *J Neurol Neurosurg Psychiatry.* 54:873.

Elwes R.D.C., Johnson A.L., Shorvon S.D., and Reynolds E.H., 1984, The prognosis for seizure control in newly diagnosed epilepsy, *N Engl J Med.* 311:944.

Gastaut, H., 1973, "Dictionary of Epilepsies. Part I: Definitions," World Health Organization, Geneva.

Goodridge D.M.G., and Shorvon S.D., 1983, Epileptic seizures in a population of 6000. II: treatment and prognosis, *Br Med J.* 287:645.

Hauser W.A., 1986, Should people be treated after a first seizure?, *Arch Neurol.* 43:1287.

Hirtz D.G., and Nelson K.B., 1985, Cognitive effects of antiepileptic drugs, in: "Recent Advances in Epilepsy 2, " T.A. Peddley and B.S. Meldrum, eds., Churchill Livingstone, Edinburgh.

Hopkins A., ed., 1987, "Epilepsy," Chapman and Hall, London.

Oller-Daurella L., and Oller Ferrer-Vidal L., 1985, "¿Qué se Puede Lograr en el Tratamiento del Epiléptico?," Geigy, Barcelona.

Oxley J., Janz D., and Meinardi H., 1983, "Chronic Toxicity of Antiepileptic Drugs," Raven Press, New York.

Porter R.J., 1984, "Epilepsy: 100 Elementary Principles," Saunders, London.

Porter R.J., 1986, Antiepileptic drugs: efficacy and inadequacy, in: "New Anticonvulsant Drugs," B.S. Meldrum and R.J. Porter, eds., John Libbey, London.

Porter R.J., 1988, New antiepileptic drugs: prospects for improved treatment of seizures, in: "Recent Advances in Epilepsy 4, " T.A. Peddley and B.S. Meldrum, eds., Churchill Livingstone, Edinburgh.

Porter R.J., and Morselli P.L., 1985, "The Epilepsies," Butterworths, London.

Reynolds E.H., 1986, Existing needs in the medical treatment of epilepsy, in: "International Workshop on Flunarizine in Epilepsy. Health Science Review," KPR, Brussels.

Rowland L.P., ed., 1989, "Merritt's Textbook of Neurology," eight edition, Lea & Febiger, Philadelphia.

Smith D.F., Baker G.A., Dewey M., et al, 1991, Seizure frequency, patient-perceived seizure severity and the psychosocial consequences of intractable epilepsy, *Epilepsy Res.* 9:231.

Van Belle G., and Temkin N.R., 1981, Design strategies in the clinical evaluation of new antiepileptic drugs, in: "Recent Advances in Epilepsy 1, " T.A: Peddley and B.S. Meldrum, eds., Churchill Livingstone, Edinburgh.

Wijsman D.J.P., Hekster Y.A., Keyser A., Renier W.O., and Meinardi H., 1991, Clinimetrics and epilepsy care, *Pharm Weekbl* [Sci]. 13:182.

QUANTITATIVE APPROACHES TO SEIZURE SEVERITY

Joyce A. Cramer, B.S. and Richard H. Mattson, M.D.

Department of Veterans Affairs Medical Center
Epilepsy Center
West Haven, Connecticut 06516, U.S.A.

INTRODUCTION

Assessment of the severity of seizures or their clinical manifestations may be of equal or greater impact on patient functional status as the total number of seizures. However, subjective and qualitative aspects of seizures are difficult to quantify. The major problems inherent in assessing seizure severity include dependence on patient recall and reporting, as well as observer documentation. Reports focus on whether the patient was alert and in control during a seizure, whether a warning aura (simple partial onset) preceded altered consciousness, whether a fall during a seizure caused self-injury (e.g., compression fracture during tonic-clonic seizures) and similar items as major issues in assessing seizure severity.

Until the early 1980's, methods of evaluation of seizure severity were largely dependent on notation of seizure type to define severity. A complex partial seizure was assumed to be more severe (i.e., diminished functional status) than a simple partial seizure. However, patient perception of seizure severity may be very different. For example, a simple partial seizure with an obvious and uncontrollable motor component could be more compromising to a patient than a brief alteration of consciousness with aphasia that is not noticed by others. Similarly, a complex partial seizure with loss of consciousness, falling, head and body turning, and urinary incontinence, is just as embarrassing and almost as likely to cause injury as a generalized tonic clonic seizure. Some patients complain about simple partial seizures because they occur with full consciousness and are noticeable to the patient, whereas some patients are totally unaware of their complex partial seizures. Effective drug therapy that reduces seizure spread resulting in simple instead of complex partial seizures may lead patients to complain or report increased seizure frequency because they have become aware of their seizures.

Quantitative Assessment in Epilepsy Care, Edited by H. Meinardi et al.
Plenum Press, New York, 1993

The evaluation of epilepsy treatment might be improved if clinical impressions could be tabulated in a standardized manner. In an early attempt to assess events, Gruber et al. (Gruber et al., 1957) graded generalized seizures as two points and focal seizures as one point, to provide an estimate of a seizure severity score over three days of observation. Cereghino et al. (Cereghino et al., 1974) equated two partial seizures with one generalized seizure using an analysis that accounted for the number of excess seizures of each seizure type. Advancing beyond seizure classification as the sole difference in severity, later investigations utilized a variety of issues that are commonly reported by patients in addition to other items that can be reported objectively. Assigning relative values to aspects of seizure severity should be based on the supposed importance of the item to the patient. For general purposes, the impact of each item on the typical epilepsy patient can be estimated using numerical scores or questions that allow patient responses to be graded.

SEIZURE SEVERITY SCALES: DESCRIPTIONS

Three scales have been developed to assess seizure severity and a fourth scale rates potential hazards causes by seizures. During the planning for the Department of Veterans Affairs (VA) Cooperative Study of Antiepileptic Drugs (Mattson et al., 1983), the need for a systematic approach to assessment of seizures led to the development of scales specific for seizure frequency and severity as well as systemic toxicity and neurotoxicity (Cramer et al., 1983). These two types of scales were combined into a single composite score that represented the overall status for the individual patient at a point in time. This approach presented a proportional consideration to the gradations in severity and frequency of seizures. Concerned with the complexity and focus of the VA rating scale, both the Chalfont (Duncan & Sander, 1991) and Liverpool (Baker et al., 1991) groups almost simultaneously proposed alternate seizure severity scales in 1991 that focus on other aspects of seizure severity. The impact of seizures on occupational suitabilities is described in an occupational hazards scale devised by Thorbecke and Janz (Janz, 1989).

VA Seizure Frequency and Severity Rating Scale

In 1978, the VA Cooperative Study Group developed a clinimetric approach to seizure assessment (Cramer et al., 1983) for use in a controlled clinical trial of antiepileptic drugs (Mattson et al., 1985). The scales were developed to provide a quantitative assessment of qualitative effects during a clinical trial that compared four standard antiepileptic drugs. The end points of the study were based on seizure counts as well as rating scale scores. The scale was slightly modified in 1985 based on initial experiences, for use in a second controlled clinical trial of antiepileptic drugs (Mattson et al., 1985) (Table 1).

The VA seizure frequency and severity rating scale was designed to combine the impact of a) type of seizures, b) number of each type of seizure, and c) factors affecting the severity of each type of seizure. Although intended only for use in evaluating simple and complex partial seizures or generalized tonic clonic seizures of primary or secondary type, the originators indicated that additional components could be developed for assessment of other types of seizures (e.g., absence, myoclonic). Each section of the rating scale is devoted to assessment of a specific type of seizure so that patients who experience multiple types of seizures can be tabulated in this three column format.

Each of these sections begins with documentation of the total number of seizures. The number of complex and simple partial seizures are tabulated since the previous visit with the physician. Because tonic-clonic seizures are relatively uncommon, the total number of the seizures since starting the drug (or some other starting point) is also listed. Seizure frequency is then graded with the number of points relative to the assumed severity of simple versus complex partial versus generalized tonic-clonic seizures. Thereafter, the scale continues with a series of questions designed to establish the relative severity of the seizures.

Modifiers of Seizure Severity

The modifiers of seizure severity included in the VA scale were selected based on clinical judgment of the most common issues used by epileptologists to assess seizure severity. The list can be expanded, deleted, or altered for any purpose.

(1) Generalized tonic-clonic and complex partial seizures are modified in severity if they begin with a simple partial seizure during which the patient is aware that an event was about to occur and can take precaution to avoid self-harm. The presence of a warning is considered to diminish the severity by twenty percent of the original score.

(2) If the patient could report that a seizure was preceded by a precipitating factor (e.g., lack of sleep, or overuse of alcohol). Other factors (e.g., an illness such as a viral infection that might diminish seizure threshold) also are common seizure precipitants. These factors are considered as reducing the impact of the seizure on normal function. Seizure score is reduced by fifty percent.

(3) If a drug level drawn soon after the seizure was below the target range for the drug, or in the low target range (as defined in the clinical trial protocol), the seizure score is decreased. This modifier is based on two factors that could have led to the seizures: a) under-prescribing by the physician, or b) under-compliance by the patient. Reducing the score prevented penalizing the drug for lack of efficacy when the seizure is more likely related to under-use of the drug. This modifier is particularly important in the context of a clinical trial to evaluate drug efficacy. Scores are reduced by seventy percent if drug levels are below the target range and twenty percent if drug levels are only in the low range.

(4) If seizures are modified by a known and highly predictable cyclic or diurnal pattern so that all seizures experienced by that patient are nocturnal or occur only during awakening, the severity is diminished. Scores are reduced by forty percent.

(5) Seizures that cause altered consciousness or significant interference with function are considered more severe than those that can be hidden from observers. The score for

Table 1. VA seizure type and frequency rating

Patient's name_____Study no._____/_____ _____
Form completed by_____ Date ____/____/____
                                                                    (Mo) (Day) (Yr)

Protocol_____type_____Drug type_____
Rating Period: 1 wk 2 wk 1 mo 2 mo 3 mo 4 mo 6 mo 9 mo 12 mo 15 mo 18 mo 21 mo 24 mo 30 mo 36 mo 42 mo
                   48 mo mo 54 mo 60 mo Unscheduled

Instructions: Record all seizures reported by patient since last visit. Use sections A, B, and C as necessary for each type of seizure reported.

Section A. GENERALIZED TONIC CLONIC SEIZURES

Complete this section if patient is either primary or secondarily generalized tonic clonic seizures.

1. Total number of seizures since last visit_____.
  Total number of seizures since start drug_____.
2. Select the seizure frequency category that applies to the patient from the following list and enter on score line.
a. Three or more seizures/12 months =   20 each seizure
(After one year review past 12 months only for multiple seizures.)

b. Two seizures/first 3 months =	50
c. Two seizures/6 months =	45

d. One seizure/first 3 months =	40
e. One seizure/6 months =	40

f. Two seizures/6-12 months =	30
g. One seizure/6-12 months =	20

h. Two seizures/12-24 months =	20
i. One seizure/12-24 months =	10

                Score_____
3. Was seizure(s) modified by an aura (allowing avoidance of harm)?
_____1. Yes ____2. No
If yes, change score to 80% of score in item 2; if no, keep score the same. Score _____
4. Was seizure(s) precipitated by unusual, remediable factors (e.g., lack of sleep, alcohol, illness)?
_____1. Yes ____2. No
If yes, change score to 50% of score in itme 3; if no, keep score the same. Score_____
5.   a. If subtherapeutic drug levels, change score to 30% of score in item 4; if not, keep the score the same.
                  Score_____
    b. If low therapeutic drug levels, change score to 80% of score in item 4; if not, keep score the same.
                  Score_____
6. Are seizures modified by known cyclic or diurnal pattern (e.g., nocturnal or early a.m.)
_____1. Yes ____2. No
If yes, change score to 60% of score in item 5; if no, keep score the same.
Generalized Tonic Clonic: Section A Final Score_____

Section B. COMPLEX PARTIAL SEIZURES

Complete this section if patient had complex partial seizures (with altered consciousness) that did not generalize.

1. Total number of seizures since last visit_____.
2. Did seizures occur as a cluster (greater than 2 seizures within 24 hours)?_____1. Yes _____2. No
    a. If yes, how many seizures occurred?_____.
    b. If three or more seizures/cluster, count only one-half the number of seizures in that cluster._____
3. Select the seizure frequency category that applies to the patient from the following list and enter on score line.

a. Equal to or greater than 4/month (+10 for each additional seizure/mo over 4)	= 50 (+10 each)
b. Equal to 3/month =	40
c. Equal to 2/month =	30
d. Equal to 1/month =	20
e. Less than 1/mo & greater than 1 per 3 mos =	15
f. Less than or equal to 1 per 3 months =	10

                Score_____
4. Was seizure(s) modified by an aura (allowing avoidance of harm)?
_____1. Yes _____2. No
If yes, change score to 80% of score in item 3; if no, keep score the same.
5. Was seizure(s) precipitated by unusual, remediable factors (e.g., lack of sleep, alcohol, illness)?
_____1. Yes _____2. No
If yes, change score to 50% of score in item 4; if no, keep score the same.
                Score_____
6. a. If subtherapeutic drug levels, change score to 30% of score in item 5; if not, keep score the same.
                Score_____
   b. If low therapeutic drug levels, change score to 80% of score in item 5; if not, keep score the same.
                Score_____
7. Are seizures modified by known cyclic and diurnal patterns (e.g., all nocturnal or early a.m.)?
_____1. Yes _____2. No
If yes, change score to 60% of score in item 6; if no, keep score the same.
                Score_____
8. Did seizure(s) cause loss of consciousness (include psychic, cognitive, and autonomic disturbances) or significant interference with functioning?
_____1. Yes _____2. No
If no, change score to 50% of score in item 7; if yes, keep score the same.

COMPLEX PARTIAL SEIZURES: Section B Final Score__

Section C. SIMPLE PARTIAL SEIZURES
Complete this section if patient had simple partial seizures
(without altered of consciousness).

1. Total number of seizure since last visit _____.
2. Did seizures occur as a cluster (greater than 2 seizures
within 24 hours)?
    _____1. Yes _____2. No
    a. If yes, how many seizures occurred?_____.
    b. If three or more seizures/cluster, count only one-half
    the number of seizures in that cluster (e.g., 6
    seizures/cluster = 3 seizures/week).
    _____ seizures/week
3. Select the seizure frequency category that applies to the
patient from the following list and enter on score line.
    a. Equal to or greater than 7/month
       (+3 for each additional
       seizure/mo over 7) =   33 (+3 each)
    b. Equal to 6/month =   30
    c. Equal to 5/month =   28
    d. Equal to 4/month =   25
    e. Equal to 3/month =   23
    f. Equal to 2/month =   20
    g. Equal to 1/month =   15
    h. Less than 1/mo & greater
       than 1 per 3 mos =   13
    i. Less than or equal 1 per 3 mos 10
           Score_____
4. Was seizure(s) precipitated by unusual, remediable factors
(e.g., lack of sleep, alcohol, illness)?
    _____1. Yes _____2. No
If yes, change score to 50% of score in item 3; if no, keep
score the same.
           Score_____

5.   a. If subtherapeutic drug levels, change score to 30% of
      score in item 4; if not, keep score the same.
           Score_____
    b. If low therapeutic drug levels, change score to 80% of
      score in item 4; if not, keep score the same.
           Score_____
6. Are seizures modified by known cyclic and diurnal patterns
(e.g., all nocturnal or early a.m.)?
    _____1. Yes _____2. No
If yes, change score to 60% of score in item 5; if no, keep
score the same.
           Score_____
7. Did seizure(s) cause significant interference with
functioning?
    _____1. Yes _____2. No
If no, change score to 50% of score in item 6; if yes, keep
score the same.

SIMPLE PARTIAL SEIZURES: Section C Final Score____

SEIZURE TYPE, FREQUENCY AND SEVERITY
RATING (sum of sections A, B, and C): Total Score____

---

milder events is reduced by fifty percent. For example, a brief alteration of awareness is considered mild, whereas a seizure with automatisms resulting in lengthy post-ictal confusion is considered more severe, although both are complex partial seizures.

VA Seizure Type and Frequency Rating

The design of the VA rating system includes emphasis on the role of antiepileptic drug treatment as much as on the occurrence of seizures. Because the scale was designed for a clinical trial comparing antiepileptic drugs, one concept was focused on evaluating the role of antiepileptic drug treatment of seizure frequency and severity. Therefore, if drug therapy was not appropriate for the individual, the seizure would have a modified score because it did not represent optimum clinical management for that patient. Similarly, precipitating factors also are remediable and unusual events, some of which can be controlled by a patient who knows that lack of sleep, or use of alcohol, will exacerbate his seizures. The rationale for designing the scale with these modifiers was based on a representation of typical clinical practice. Physicians who hear of a seizure breakthrough related to a precipitating factor or known non-compliance usually are less likely to alter the treatment plan than if the patient is at an optimal status with drug dose and levels relative to adverse effects.

Wijsman et al. (1991) validated the VA scale during an assessment of the practicability of clinimetric indexes in clinical care. Consistency and suitability were evaluated statistically. Consistency was tested by Spearman correlation coefficients for 24 paired scores. Monitor and evaluator scores correlated well (r = 0.90). Inter-rater agreement between experienced epileptologists and untrained neurologists was 67% (Kappa = 0.52).

The VA scale is not an overall quality of life measure, although is does represent the patient's perspective of the impact of seizures on his normal function to some extent. Other than the modifying question for complex and simple partial seizures related to altered consciousness and interference with functioning, the items approach the effectiveness of antiepileptic drug therapy rather than patient function. In these clinical trials, it was most important to develop a standardized basis of optimizing drug therapy for all patients before evaluating comparisons among drugs. In the VA system, the seizure score is added to adverse effect scores, providing a composite score that represents overall patient status. A difference of approximately 10 points in the *composite score* reflects a clinically important difference as judged by epileptologists.

Chalfont Seizure Severity Scale

The Chalfont Seizure Severity Scale (Duncan & Sander, 1991), like the VA scale, uses both patient information and observer interpretations for the ratings. The simple format of the scale is further explained in appendix notes that provide instructions for completion of each item. Columns are provided for up to three types of seizures without notation of the frequency of seizures. The scale provides a variety of seizure severity items, most of which are parallel to questions in the VA scale. As with all rater based scales, the reliability depends on the quality of information reported by the patient and observers. Inter-rater and test-retest reliability were assessed by interviewing patients and reliable observers, repeated within 2–3 weeks (Duncan & Sander, 1991). Two observers evaluated 93 seizures in 57 patients, resulting in an inter-rater coefficient of reliability of 13.4; test-retest reliability was 15.9 for 101 seizures in 34 patients. No relationships were found between the mean of the observer scores and the difference between scores.

As illustrated in Table 2, the first two items (describing loss of awareness and a warning) represent differences between simple and complex partial seizures. Dropping or spilling liquids and falling to the ground describe interference with function. The items stipulating injury and incontinence are important issues for severity rating that are pertinent to generalized tonic-clonic seizures as well as severe complex partial seizures. Differences in automatisms, ranging from mild to severe, more clearly define interference with function. Occurrence of a convulsion or generalized tonic-clonic seizure is documented separately. Both the duration of the seizure and the time to return to normal are categorized to define point scores related to relative interference with function. The items defining time/span are important issues of severity for the patient whose lengthy seizure or post-ictal period usually cannot be camouflaged. Points are apportioned based on the number of times each modifier occurred in the overall number of seizures. Nocturnal seizures require a simple modification of fifty percent reduction in score. The Chalfont scale weights the duration of impaired consciousness as the most important aspect of altered function for the patient. Nevertheless, the authors disclaim the role of the Chalfont scale as an overall measure of epilepsy or overall functional status. It is designed for use in longitudinal evaluations of individual patients in clinical practice or clinical trials.

Liverpool Seizure Severity Scale

The Liverpool group (Baker et al., 1991) developed a mode to assess seizure frequency, patient perceived seizure severity, and psychosocial consequences of intractable epilepsy. The 19 items in the seizure severity scale, an integral part of the model, (Table 3) are answered by the patient without interpretation by the health care provider and represent seizure activity during the previous four weeks. The scale is divided into two sections, one reviewing perceptions of control and the other reviewing ictal and post-ictal effects. The scale is self-administered to allow patients to report their perceptions rather than have the health care provider evaluate severity for that individual. Baker et al. (1991) report the test-retest reliability and validity of the scale (by comparing patients with different seizure types). The scale does not differentiate perception of control by seizure type but does reflect seizure severity effects. The scale items serve as descriptions of the patient's perception of the impact of seizures on daily function without assigning points for each item. This format does not provide information about the exact number of seizures nor does this scale describe specific seizure classification which would have to be documented by an epileptologist. The Liverpool scale is designed to evaluate individual seizure types, not the overall severity of epilepsy. A suggested use is to measure change of severity of partial seizures. Additional studies are ongoing to incorporate the seizure severity scales within a quality of life scale to assess the overall impact of epilepsy on patient function.

Test-retest reliability (Pearson correlation coefficient) was 0.8 for the ictal/post-ictal scale and 0.79 for the percept scale, confirming consistency overtime. Internal consistencies were 0.85 and 0.69 respectively, as the Cronbach alpha score. Pearson correlations between patients and their relatives or carers were 0.64 to 0.77 for four items drawn from the scale.

Occupational Hazard Scale

Janz (1989) considered the taxonomy of seizure classification less important to the patient than the possible social impairment caused by a seizure (e.g., maintaining posture instead of falling reduces the risk of accidents). They used the scale to evaluate the suitability of patients for selected occupations based on the severity of their seizures. The seven item scale (Table 4) gives examples of types of seizures and treatment status. Seizure-free patients who qualify for driver's license are least affected, and those whose seizures are frequent, include falling, or impair activity, are most impaired. Although the scale describes only a small number of possible examples, it can serve as a guide for grading occupational suitability or changes in patient status over time if seizure severity changes.

Table 2. Chalfont seizure severity scale[a]

Classification of Seizure Types	Seizures		
	Type 1	Type 2	Type 3
Loss of awareness no = 0, yes = 1			
Warning (if loss of awareness) no = 1, yes = 0			
Drop, spill a held object no = 0, yes = 4			
Fall to ground no = 0, yes = 4			
Injury no = 0, yes = 20			
Incontinent no = 0, yes = 8			
Automatism no = 0 mild (chew, swallow, fiddle) = 4 severe (shout, undress, run, hit) = 12			
Convulsion no = 0, yes = 12			
Duration of seizure <10 sec = 0, 10 sec-1 min = 1 1-10 min = 4, >10 min = 16			
Time to return to normal from onset <1 min = 0, 1-10 min = 5, 10-30 min = 20 30-60 min = 30, 1-3 hr = 50, >3 hr = 100			
If epileptic event (e.g., brief aura) with total score = 0, then add 1			
Divide score by 2 if seizures are only in sleep			
TOTAL SCORE			

Appendix Notes on Completion of Chalfont Seizure Severity Scale

1) Classification of seizure type, according to International League against Epilepsy Classification

2) In each section, score what usually occurs in that seizure type with fractionation as follows; No score if that factor does not occur; Quarter score if occurs in up to 25% of occurrences; Half score if occurs in 25%-50% of occurrences; Three quarters score if occurs in 50%-75% of occurrences; Full score if occurs in >75% of occurrences; For example, if injury in 50%-75% of occurrences, injury score = 15. If dropping a held object in up to 25% of occurrences, dropping a held object score = 1. Scores for loss of awareness and warning to a seizure are not amenable to fractionation.

3) Drop, spill a held object includes spilling a held drink, even if the vessel is not dropped.

4) Injury includes tongue-biting, bruising and lacerations.

5) Incontinence includes urine and faeces.

6) Automatism. Mild implies features that are not socially disabling, for example, chewing, repeated swallowing, fiddling with objects. Severe implies features that are socially disabling, such as swearing, running, undressing, hitting out. This score may also be fractionated (see note 2, above).

7) Convulsion is taken to mean clonic jerking of limbs.

8) Duration of seizure. Time from onset, until judged to have terminated, by patient and/or a reliable witness.

9) Time to return to normal from onset is taken as the duration of time until the patient is able to resume the activity that they were pursuing when the seizure occurred.

10) A score of 1 is added, if the total score otherwise = 0. For example a simple partial seizure consisting of an epigastric rising sensation that lasts less than 10 seconds.

11) If a given seizure type occurs only in sleep, the total score, for that seizure type is divided by 2.

12) The total of the scores obtained for a given seizure type is its severity score.

[a] Reproduced with permission from Duncan and Sander, 1991.

Table 3. Liverpool seizure severity scale items[a]

PERCEPTION ITEMS

1. Time of day of seizure occurrence (day or night)
2. Ability to predict seizure occurrence
3. Ability to abort ("fight off") seizures
4. Presence of a warning or simple partial seizure (aura) preceding some or all attacks
5. Perception of control over attacks
6. Clustering of seizures
7. Frequency of nocturnal seizures
8. Degree of seizure interference with daily function (lifestyle)
9. Severity of seizure
10. Duration of altered consciousness   **ICTAL/POST ICTAL ITEMS**
11. Degree of post-ictal confusion
12. Duration of post-ictal confusion
13. Falling during a seizure
14. Frequency of post-ictal headache
15. Frequency of post-ictal sedation
16. Frequency of urinary incontinence
17. Frequency of tongue biting
18. Frequency of self-injury related to a seizure
19. Duration of altered function after a seizure

[a] Adapted with permission from Baker, 1991.

Table 4. Occupational hazard scale[a]

TYPE OF SEIZURES TREATMENT STATUS	OCCUPATIONAL HAZARD	#
Seizure free (allowed to drive motor vehicle)		1
Seizures only during sleep not more than 1/month Unilateral jerks without loss of consciousness not more than 1/week		2
Seizures only during sleep not more than 1/week Very brief seizures impairing or interrupting ongoing activity not more than 1/six months		3
Brief seizures impairing or interrupting ongoing activity not more than 1/six months Unilateral jerks without loss of consciousness Seizures with falling lasting less than 5 min including reorientation not more than 1/six months		4
Seizures during which person does not behave according to demands of situation not more than 1/month Seizures with falling lasting less than 15 min including reorientation not more than 1/month		5
Seizures impairing or interrupting ongoing activity Seizures during which person does not behave according to demands of situation not more than 1/week Seizures with falling lasting less than 15 min not more than 1/week		6

[a] Adapted from Janz,1989, with permission.

Seizure Severity Items: Use in Each Scale

Evaluation of seizure severity includes many issues, each of which is used in one or more of the scales. Many of these topics are difficult for the patient to describe because of lack of recall, absence of an observer, or infrequency of events so the patient is not aware of the relationship of the event to seizure (e.g., olfactory aura as a sensory component of a seizure). Even when a patient cannot recall the clinical details or duration of a seizure, he or she can report whether it caused embarrassment or self-harm. Patients also commonly recall associated precipitating factors that they relate to seizure occurrence. Rather than attempting to document all clinical details of seizures, as can be done during inpatient closed-circuit television monitoring, an outpatient self-report system must be based on information that the patients can recall and describe. In the following sections, each component of seizure severity is described and its use in each scale is mentioned. Table 5 lists the 13 items used in at least one of the scales, with much similarly among the approaches to seizure severity issues.

1. Seizure Type

Patients who recognize the presence of a sensation or movement typical of their simple partial seizures can report these events. Sensory and motor activities occurs alone or previous to altered consciousness during the progression to a complex partial seizure. Not only is a simple partial seizure less severe than one during which consciousness is altered, but also the progression from a simple partial to a complex partial seizure alerts the patient and serves as a warning to sit down, stop driving, or halt other activities that would lead to harmful sequelae if consciousness were altered. Individual patients can recognize the intensity of their simple partial seizure and the likely progression to a complex partial event.

The VA scale used lowest scores for simple partial seizures, slightly higher scores for complex partial seizures, and the highest penalty scores for generalized tonic clonic seizures to account for the gradations in seizure severity. The Chalfont scale reflects seizure type as a measure of severity by scoring 12 points for convulsions, and allowing one point for brief simple partial seizures (auras). Falling to the ground also may be considered as aspect of seizure type (4 points). The Liverpool scale provides columns for major and minor seizures to represent seizure type. The Occupational Hazard scale does not address seizure type. The scales have similar approaches to seizure severity by seizure type.

2. Seizure Duration

The duration of seizures, particularly complex partial seizures that have lengthy post-ictal periods of impaired function clearly affect the patient's perception of the severity of

Table 5. Seizure severity items used in scales

1. Seizure type	8. Stopping seizures
2. Seizure duration	9. Tongue biting and incontinence
3. Post-ictal events and duration	10. Other injuries
4. Automatisms	11. Precipitating factors
5. Seizure clusters	12. Drug levels and compliance
6. Cyclic and diurnal patterns	13. Functional impairment
7. Prediction of seizures	

the event. Brief absence or simple partial seizures can be hidden from observers, but a lengthy complex partial seizure followed by twenty minutes of aphasia and cognitive impairment will be highly noticeable. Not only is a long seizure obvious to an observer, but it also requires precautions to avoid harm particularly when driving and working. Patients who know that their seizures are always brief can take more risks than patients of whom seizures are sometimes or often lengthy.

The VA scale does not consider seizure duration. The Chalfont scale scores an increasing number of points depending on the duration of the seizure, up to 16 points. The Liverpool scale rates the duration of altered consciousness and post-ictal confusion as well as the total duration of time during which the patient is affected by the seizure. The Occupational Hazard scale considers brevity of seizures.

3. Post-ictal Events and Duration

For many patients, a brief seizure is followed by a lengthy period of post-ictal confusion or sedation. The patient perceives the ictal and post-ictal phases of a seizure as a continuum, caring little for the electro-clinical definitions that separate these phases of a seizure. Seizure severity can be graded on the duration of the post-ictal events, the type of phenomena (e.g., aphasia, sedation, confusion).

The VA scale does not consider the post-ictal period. The Chalfont scale scores increasing numbers of points depending on the specific duration of time until return to normal functions (up to 100 points). The Liverpool scale questions both the degree and severity of post-ictal confusion. The Occupational Hazard scale considers frequency of impaired function and brevity of seizures.

4. Automatisms

Seizures that include automatic behaviour during periods of altered consciousness are highly visible to observers who recognize that the patient is not acting normally. Chewing or swallowing facial movement may be ignored but seeing a patient speak loudly or incoherently, undress, or run away is clearly aberrant behaviour. The perceived severity of an automatism in terms of its social acceptability or ability of the patient to hide the automatism also is an aspect of functional impairment related to seizure severity. Some automatisms with obvious physical impairment can be deterrents to patients' ability to drive, work, or be out in public alone.

The VA scale does not separate the presence of automatisms from the overall severity of complex partial seizures but allows for score reduction if the features of the seizure (e.g., automatisms) are not bothersome to the patient under the category of functional impairment. The Chalfont scale specifies types of mild automatisms (e.g., chew, swallow) that are usually not noticed by other people (4 points) and severe automatisms (e.g., shout, undress) that are noticeably and embarrassing to the patient (12 points). The Liverpool scale does not address automatisms. The Occupational Hazard scale describes unusual behaviour.

5. Seizure Clusters

Although a patient can experience multiple seizures in a cluster, the impact on function is modified by the clustering phenomena. Those patients who know that when they have seizures, all events will occur over a period of a few hours or days can be comfortable driving and working at other times. Clustering of seizures is further mitigated if a known cyclic pattern is common for the individual (e.g., during menses).

The VA scale includes a mechanism to reduce seizure severity by counting only half of the seizures occurring in a cluster. The Chalfont scale does not include this issue. The Liverpool scale asks about the likelihood that seizures occur in clusters. The Occupational Hazard scale does not consider seizure clusters.

6. Cyclic or Diurnal Patterns

Some fortunate patients have seizures only at night or in the early morning during awakening. This is an advantage over the usually sporadic occurrence of seizures because these patients know that once they are fully awake and alert, they can drive and work without fear of a seizure during the day. This characteristic is helpful to the patient only if it is consistent with all seizures occurring into the expected pattern. All three of the seizure severity scales include this item.

The VA scales reduce scores by 40%. The Chalfont scale allows for score reduction by half for nocturnal seizures. The Liverpool scale asks both about the usual time of day when seizures occur and whether seizures occur nocturnally. Both question relates to lesser severity if the patient knows when to expect seizures. The Occupational Hazard scale considers the frequency of nocturnal seizures.

7. Prediction of Seizures

In addition to known cyclic or diurnal patterns, some patients are able to predict when they will have seizures based on known precipitants. Most patient reports of ability to predict when seizures will occur are probably the sensations or motor activity related to simple partial seizures that warn the individual of impending complex partial or generalized tonic-clonic seizures, particularly if the simple partial events occur serially.

The VA scale does not address this issue. This modifier is addressed in the Chalfont scale with a one point penalty for seizures without warning before loss of awareness. The Liverpool scale rates the likelihood that the patient could predict a seizure. The Occupational Hazard scale does not address prediction of seizures.

8. Stopping Seizures

A number of patients report an ability to abort seizures by using a variety of mental and physical tactics, most commonly including mental concentration. This type of self-report probably relates to feeling simple partial seizures that are prevented from spreading to cause altered consciousness. The technique of biofeedback has been used for many years to teach patients how to concentrate and recruit alpha waves to abort seizures or prevent spread. Only the Liverpool scale asks whether and how often the patient "fights off attacks."

9. Tongue Biting and Incontinence

Although both tongue biting and incontinence are often considered the hallmarks of a generalized tonic-clonic seizure, urinary incontinence also occurs with severe complex partial seizures. In addition, urinary (and particularly faecal) incontinence can cause extreme embarrassment. Tongue biting is often noticed by observers after the patient has recovered from the seizure. The VA scale does not separate these features from the overall severity of tonic clonic seizures. The Chalfont scale scores eight points for incontinence only. The Liverpool scale asks about both tongue biting and urinary incontinence. The Occupational Hazard scale does not address these issues.

10. Other Injuries

Whether or not the seizure is a generalized tonic-clonic seizure or a complex partial seizure with altered consciousness or other type of generalized seizure disorder involving loss of muscle tone, seizures that include falling are severe in their likelihood of causing bodily harm and social ostracism. Self-injury during a seizure is not uncommon during generalized tonic-clonic seizures. Patients often suffer broken teeth, cuts, bruises, burns, and bone fractures, including thoracic vertebrae. The VA scale does not address this issue. Chalfont scale scores 20 points for injury. The Liverpool scale asks about the likelihood of self-injury and falling to the ground. The Occupational Hazard scale emphasizes the possibility of injury related to seizures.

11. Remediable Precipitating Factors

Patients frequently report remediable precipitating factors that preceded their seizures. Common examples are lack of sleep, or use of alcoholic beverages. Patients whose seizures are susceptible to change in sleep, or alcohol thresholds are told (or must learn from experience) about the importance of avoiding these precipitants. By reporting occurrence of one or more precipitating factor, the patient recognizes the association between the event and the seizure. For many patients, avoidance of known precipitants will allow them to remain seizure-free. The VA scale reduced scores by 50% in the presence of remediable precipitating factors. The other scales do not include this issue.

12. Drug Levels and Compliance

Similar to precipitating factors, patients often can report that they had forgotten to take one or more doses of their antiepileptic drugs before a seizure occurred (Cramer

1991b). This information is important in evaluating the patients status because, in some respects, it documents the efficacy of the patient's current drug regimen when it is taken properly. Seizures that occur after missed doses represent a sensitive threshold to drug effects for that individual (i.e., the drug is effective when serum concentrations are maintained at a level determined to be optimum for that patient). The VA scale allows for reduction of the seizure score by 20% if levels were low or by 70% if levels were subtherapeutic. The purpose is to avoid penalizing drug efficacy when the seizure was more likely related to the patient omitting doses, or underprescribing by the physician.

Knowledge of the exact drug serum concentration at the time of the seizure is rarely available. Even if patients are requested to have a blood level test after their next seizure, many patients take their next dose immediately after the seizure, before having the blood test. If the blood level soon after the seizure is known, this information allows the physician to evaluate modifications in drug therapy in hopes of preventing further seizures. A second aspect of using drug levels in assessing seizure severity is compliance (Cramer, 1991a). If the patient can recall having forgotten a dose (even if no drug level is available), the assumption can be made that the steady-state drug serum concentrations were lower than usual at the time of the seizure. Unfortunately, studies of epilepsy patients have demonstrated that patients frequently are unaware that they have forgotten one or more doses. Patient inability to report this information and lack of a recent drug level make it difficult for a clinician to assess the need to adjust the antiepileptic drug regimen after a seizure occurs.

The recent development of microelectronic monitoring techniques provide specific information about patient dosing habits including the number of doses taken daily, the time of the dose, and the interval between doses (Cramer et al., 1989). A review of these data shows whether the patient has a typical regimen of taking doses at approximately the same time each day, with or without alterations on weekends or during vacation periods (Cramer et al., 1990). If the patient can report the date of a seizure, rapid scan of the microelectronic monitoring data will show the physician whether missed doses were a likely precipitant for this seizure. In addition, a review of the number of doses taken on several days preceding the seizure will suggest whether steady-state drug levels might have dropped (e.g., if only one dose was taken daily for the week before the seizure instead of the prescribed two doses, steady-state drug levels probably were half what was expected). The dosing calendar also will demonstrate whether dosing was omitted over several days before a seizure, whereas missing an occasional dose did not result in a seizure. These several levels of information provide important information about the likely seizure threshold and sensitivity to changes in drug levels for the individual patient who has occasional seizures.

13. Functional Impairment

Even simple partial seizures can cause a significant interference with normal functioning, particularly if multiple seizures occur serially. For example, a patient may be able to hide one or two simple partial seizures but will be noticeably affected by co-workers when several seizures occur. Complex partial seizures that include psychic or cognitive disturbances are readily apparent to observers who view the patient acting strangely. In addition to social effects, the patient's ability to drive or work often is impaired, which could lead to self-harm. Thus, the level of functional interference of simple or complex partial seizures is related to the severity of the seizures.

The VA scale allows for mild simple and complex partial seizures which do not interfere with function to be scored at 50% of the standard score. The Chalfont scale item for automatisms can be considered to reflect functional impairment with scores of 4 points for mild automatism and 12 points for socially unacceptable automatisms. The Liverpool scale specifically asks about seizure interference with daily function in terms of the patient's ability to do all of the things he or she "wants to do." The Occupational Hazard scale considers frequency and duration of impaired function.

COMPARISON AMONG SCALES

While the four published seizure severity rating scales are quite similar in the type of items considered to assess seizure severity, none includes all of the items. The difference between a patient questionnaire and a health care provider completed format also alters the type of information collected.

Scales of these types are particularly useful in longitudinal studies in which patients can be followed over the course of time so the point scores represent changes in the overall effect of epilepsy on a patient's lifestyle. The clinimetric approach combined with a longitudinal implementation is an excellent format for use in clinical trials where various therapies (e.g., surgery or other treatment) or medication changes (investigational drugs or comparisons between drugs), can be made longitudinally.

Acknowledgment. Supported by the Department of Veterans Affairs Medical Research Service, Cooperative Studies Program.

REFERENCES

1. Baker GA, Smith DF, Dewey M, Morrow J, Crawford PM, Chadwick DW. The development of a seizure severity scale as an outcome measure in epilepsy. Epilepsy Res 1991; 8:245–251.

2. Cereghino JJ, Brock JT, Van Meter JC, Penry JK, Smith LD, White BG. Carbamazepine for epilepsy: A controlled prospective evaluation. Neurology 1974; 24:401–410.

3. Cramer JA. Overview of methods to measure and enhance patient compliance. In: Cramer JA, Spilker B, eds. Patient Compliance in Medical Practice and Clinical Trials, New York: Raven Press, 1991a; 3–10.

4. Cramer JA, Mattson RH. Monitoring compliance with antiepileptic drug therapy. In: Cramer JA, Spilker B, eds. Patient Compliance in Medical Practice and Clinical Trials, New York: Raven Press, 1991b; 1–26.

5. Cramer JA, Mattson RH, Prevey ML, Scheyer R, Ouellette V. How often is medication taken as prescribed? A novel assessment technique. JAMA 1989; 261:3273–3277.

6. Cramer JA, Scheyer R, Mattson RH. Compliance declines between clinic visits. Arch Intern Med 1990; 150:1509–1510.

7. Cramer JA, Smith DB, Mattson RH, et al. A method of quantification for the evaluation of antiepileptic drug therapy. Neurology 1983; 33:26–37.

8. Duncan JS, Sander JWAS. The Chalfont Seizure Severity Scale. J Neurol Neurosurg Psychiatry 1991; 54:873–876.

9. Gruber C, Mosier J, Grant P. Objective comparison of primidone and phenobarbital in epileptics. J Pharmacol Exp Ther 1957; 120:184–187.

10. Janz D. How does one assess the severity of epilepsy? In: Trimble MR, ed. Chronic Epilepsy: Its Prognosis and Management, New York: John Wyllie, 1989; 21–36.

11. Mattson RH, Cramer JA, Collins JF, et al. Comparison of carbamazepine, phenobarbital,phenytoin, and primidone in partial and secondary generalized tonic-clonic seizures. N Engl J Med 1985; 313: 145–151.

12. Mattson RH, Cramer JA, Escueta AVD, et al. A design for the prospective evaluation of the efficacy and toxicity of antiepileptic drugs in adults. Neurology 1983; 33:14–25.

13. Mattson RH, Cramer JA, and the VA Epilepsy Cooperative Study Group. Valproate for treatment of partial and secondarily generalized tonic-clonic seizures in adults: a comparison with carbamazepine.(in press)

14. Wijsman DJP, Hekster YA, Renier WO, Meinardi H. Clinimetrics and epilepsy care. Pharm Weekbl [sci] 1991; 13:182–188.

GENERAL DISCUSSION OF THE ASSESSMENT AND REPRESENTATION OF THE ELEMENTS SEIZURE FREQUENCY AND SEIZURE SEVERITY

MENDONÇA: When we are constructing scales we must decide on their various objectives; what is the role and function the scale is going to play? Do we intend to use a severity scale on its own, or do we want a seizure severity scale to be used as a component of a model to assess the severity of epilepsy? Seizure severity has a different meaning for patients and doctors. While neurologists emphasize the clinical and electroencephalographic manifestations as clinical markers, the patients emphasize some of the clinical aspects they are aware of and those with greater impact on their quality of life (QOL). Which of these concepts are we going to use? Which is the definition of seizure severity we are going to measure? Do we want a scale based only on clinical judgments or do we want a severity scale to measure patient's perception of severity? Can we decide upon a scale that can be used in various contexts, or has each of the available scales (VA, Chalfont, Liverpool) its own objective and its own role to play?

Furthermore Dr. Baker raised the question of how much can the patient's perception of severity be used to assess the treatment efficacy? The problem is that we know that patient's perception of severity is a difficult and especially complex issue. We have cultural, social, professional, familiar factors, but on top of that we have the individual personality traits of the patient and, as was mentioned, medical assessment is not always the same as the patient's assessment.

I would like to raise another question: is the Liverpool scale a seizure severity scale or is it an Epilepsy Severity scale by itself?

We should also discuss the scope of the seizure severity scales on the basis of seizure frequency. While the Liverpool scale points towards more severe cases of epilepsy (deals with the seizure which occurred in the previous 4 week period) the VA scale may be applied to mild/moderate epilepsy. Where is the scale going to be applied: in routine clinical practice, in routine neurological practice, in a hospital with an epilepsy unit, or in an epilepsy centre?

Very often the Glasgow Coma scale as well as the Apgar Score are referred to as good examples of easily administered and universally used scales. These scales have been constructed by clinicians and are based on clinical judgments of objective clinical characteristics of the head trauma patient and of the newborn baby. When we evaluate the score of the Glasgow Coma Scale we are concerned with severity of the trauma at a specific point in time; we are not evaluating the impact of the trauma on the life and social well-

Quantitative Assessment in Epilepsy Care, Edited by H. Meinardi et al.
Plenum Press, New York, 1993

73

being of the patient. To try to approach other aspects we have other scales such as the Karnofsky scale, but again they are concerned with physical outcome and not with variables related to intellectual and social domains. The outcome of a trauma patient will depend in part on other characteristics, such as the locus of the lesion, characteristics of the patient, age, social and cultural environment and, to a certain extent, on the availability of resources to provide the care needed.

When evaluating the Glasgow scores the patient is present, and as the score is based on objective items, no problems arise with the reliability and accuracy of the data. On the contrary when classifying the severity of a seizure based on the information recalled by the patients, problems with the accuracy of the data are of the utmost importance. As it has been mentioned there are many characteristics of a seizure the patient is not aware of and even when an observer is present at the time of the seizure some of its characteristics may be hidden from the patient for social or emotional reasons. Epilepsy is a chronic brain disorder characterized by recurrent seizures.

A scale to describe a patient's single state in time may not always be suitable for discriminating changes. Do we have to develop an index that discriminates which information can be recalled and/or gathered accurately? Are there any factors describing a seizure that can be used to assess its severity in a consistent objective way? If so, could these factors be included in a scale that could be universally used and accepted? These factors have to be easily assessed and should not be restricted by severity of the seizure as perceived by the patient or his ability to recall these factors. Could VA scale items be factors to be included in such a scale? Probably some do, but are they sufficient to describe the severity of a seizure? Is such an evaluation based solely on clinical judgment sufficiently useful in assessing the severity of a seizure when evaluating a treatment effect?

If the objective of the scale is to evaluate the seizure severity as perceived by the patients as part of a QOL index and to assess the overall impact of epilepsy on the life of the patient, would a patient-based scale be more appropriate? Problems with reliability and accuracy of the data are of the greatest concern, but should we seek an answer for those items that the patient is not aware of, i.e. based on what really happened, or only an answer based on what the patient thought that happened?

Scales have to be easily usable but also valid and reliable. Seizure severity scales, although based on objective characteristics and consequences of the seizures, incorporate many subjective issues, e.g., the Chalfont scale that measures the components of a seizure that produce most disturbances for the patients. The decision which items are important and the decision about their weights are derived from a representative sample of the typical epileptic population and may depend on cultural and socio-economic factors. The attributable importance of an item may vary dependent on culture, on the fraction of the population within the same culture, or even may vary with time. Thus these scales may be valid and reliable within a certain population, but the results may be restricted to the particular time and population that produced the data. Can scales such as these be straightforwardly applied and used within a different target population beyond the particular locale of the field study? Probably they should be adapted and the items and weights appropriately revised. Nevertheless the methodology applied to the construction of such a scale may be applied to different target populations and probably we will end up with different but similar scales.

If we think of a seizure severity scale as a component of an epilepsy severity index to evaluate the efficacy of an anti-epileptic treatment, should this scale include only items referring to the characteristics of the seizures, or should it also include items referring to possible consequences of the seizure, which may be influenced by external factors? For example in the Chalfont scale "injury" is one item which heavily influences the total score. This consequence of the seizure may be avoidable if somebody is with the patient and then the total Chalfont score will be lower. Nevertheless the characteristics of the seizure (such as loss of muscle tone) will remain the same, whether or not an injury has occurred.

After deciding which items should be included in a scale, we should look at the actual construction. In presently available scales like the Liverpool scale or the Chalfont scale (unless a given seizure type occurs only in sleep) the contribution of each item to the total score is independent of the remaining items, but in the VA-scale there are hierarchies and multiplication factors: the contribution of each item is variable (i.e., depends on the presence or absence of the characteristics of the previous seizures addressed in the scale). Would seizure severity be better expressed as a sum of scores of individual items or as an interaction between the several items?

KEYSER: Dr. Cramer is it true that your seizure scale is essentially a seizure severity scale?

CRAMER: We titled the scale "seizure type and frequency severity rating scale," because it encompasses several factors and not only one. By dividing up the specific types of seizures which we were anticipating for this particular population we made some gradations in the sense that we specifically categorised seizure frequency, which is what you are addressing, by assigning point scores based on the seizure type, and we very carefully attempted to define frequency as the basis for the initial score. We then went on to seizure severity.

As for the seizure frequency rating: this is based on a score system of 0–50 points. Of course there are no negative points for not having seizures; that simply is 0. Patients certainly could have more than 50 points if they had more seizures, but 50 was considered our "clinical sensibility" scale and at that point clinical judgment would agree with the score, that a patient probably needed a change. You might call it therefore a failure scale in the sense that if one simply uses the seizure frequency aspect of this scale and looks at the range of points from 0–50, you can say that a particular treatment has failed or not failed or needs some type of adjustment.

RENIER: Everybody says we count frequencies of seizures, but how do we count them? We cannot base our counting on diaries from the patients, certainly not for complex partial seizures. These counts are not sufficiently reliable. I think we have to propose different accounting methods for different seizure types.

CRAMER: In many cases all we have is what the patient can tell us. Unfortunately we cannot video the patients continuously and we have only this subjective assessment. Interestingly, in some studies of patients who have numerous seizures (e.g. Lennox-Gastaut or childhood absence epilepsy) an arrangement was made that the family would really observe the child for one hour after dinner, say from 6:00–7:00 pm every day, and count the seizures in that hour. Whether it was an extrapolation, or a window on the number of seizures, at least that was a clear index of what that patient was doing over time.

JOHNSON: There are a number of issues that I must raise from a statistical viewpoint with respect to seizure frequency as a treatment effect parameter. The singular most important issue is that we must have randomized studies to derive conclusions about treatments. You cannot select a group of patients on the basis that they have a seizure frequency above a specific cut-off point. Subsequently put them on treatments, observe their seizure frequency again, look at the change and interpret that as a treatment effect. Your expectation is that in the complete absence of a treatment effect, you will see a reduction in seizure frequency, produced by a statistical artifact known as regression to the mean. It is vital that that is controlled for, and for that control, you need randomization. The second point that was made was the question of looking at change in seizure frequency. There is nothing wrong with that when using randomized studies, but there are far more efficient methods of analysis than those based on simple change. The point is that you can look at your seizure frequency in the treatment periods and make comparisons, however, adjusting for the baseline seizure frequency using analysis of covariance. That is much more efficient than relying upon change by itself and could lead to reductions in numbers of patients needed in the study of the order of about thirty to forty percent. The last issue is that of creating study groups which are homogeneous for seizure frequency. You would need to put the few patients with a seizure frequency of say fifty seizures per month into a trial for many years. At the end of that period we will be able to generalize the conclusions of that study only to patients who have perhaps between forty-five and fifty-five seizures per month. We need large samples in clinical trials, we need those patients to be representative of the broad population of patients as a whole, and we should be looking for heterogeneous groups of patients and not homogeneous groups.

KEYSER: According to the studies from Baker and Smith frequency had remarkably less influence than seizure severity. I should like to ask Baker to comment on this and I should like him to include in his discussion the paper of Dr. Martins da Silva. He also applied a seizure severity scale—the Chalfont scale—and although this scale remained on the same level, the seizure frequency varied a lot in the same patients. So I think we should concentrate a bit on the phenomenon that seizure severity is experienced by the patients in a certain way and seems to be rather independent from seizure frequency.

BAKER: You are referring to a study my colleagues and I conducted over a year ago. What we looked at was 100 patients with chronic epilepsy. This was a group that was resistant to AED treatment and was being considered for surgery. These patients had a significant amount of seizures and in that study, what we attempted to do was look at the frequency and the type of seizures they were having and it's relationship to their psychological well-being. So we used a number of well validated and standardized measures of anxiety, depression, self-esteem, mastery and affect balance, and we carried out a number of multiple regression analyses, looking at the psychological factors as dependent variables and the influence of severity and frequency on them. It was clear from our results that the severity of those seizures showed a greater significant relationship to the psychological well-being than the actual frequency. Clearly the percentage variance we are talking about is small, because the factors that accounted for most of the psychological variation were other psychological variables.

It is important to note that we were looking at a group of patients with chronic intractable epilepsy. I am sure that when you are having many seizures, frequency may become less important than actual severity. We are at present conducting a survey of over 1000 patients in the Mersey region and we shall be able to tell you with that sort of range of clientele how the influence of frequency and severity each contributes to psychological well-being.

MENDONÇA: One should bear in mind that identical seizures may have a different impact on two different patients, and in addition these identical seizures may be perceived by the same patient as having different levels of severity at different points in time. First seizures may be very distressing for a patient, who may change his way of life to adapt to the seizures and subsequent seizures therefore may be perceived as less severe. On the other hand in patients with intractable epilepsy similar seizures may be perceived as more severe when the patient, aware of the persistence of his seizures and suffering from side effects of the treatment, reaches a stage of bad social adjustment.

In a patient-based scale the items and their weights are defined by a group of patients and may differ from the ones an individual patient would have emphasized if asked for his own evaluation. We may be able to use the results of the scale derived from the group-defined characteristics when comparing the efficacy of different treatments in a drug trial because we are concerned with the results for the typical epileptic population. However, in clinical practice, how could we base our judgments on a scale's score for an individual patient in order to make a decision about the most appropriate treatment for that specific patient as his individual assessment of the weight of the items may differ from that of the typical population?

BAKER: It seems to me there is room for both a physician-based and a patient-based seizure severity scale. I don't believe that the scales we have at the moment can be used for both. We developed the Liverpool scale as a patient-based scale. We have not inserted clinical information because what we are interested in primarily is what the patients perceive as the severity of their seizure.

CRAMER: I think a patient-based scale may be useful in clinical practice. The uses for a patient-based and physician-based scale are entirely different which I think all will agree.

PORTER: Do you think it's possible to have a meaningful seizure severity scale in a treatment trial, that is to say, without having an adequate documentation of seizure frequency and only the patient's information about the severity?

CRAMER: I quite agree with the point of your question and the answer is no. I would not think that they can be separated.

MEINARDI: Dr. Baker, does the Liverpool scale represent epilepsy control?

BAKER: We certainly did include the perception of control. I would, however, not describe the Liverpool scale as an epilepsy scale, because there are some important issues that are missing from it.

MENDONCA: Can that scale be used in clinical practice to make a clinical judgment about treatment?

BAKER: We actually used it in a double-blind cross-over study comparing an add-on anti-epileptic drug with placebo. In clinical practice it would be of interest to use it for assessing the disability of an individual. In its present form its use is rather restricted, however.

MEINARDI: In the course of some other discussions the question was raised whether the Liverpool scale suffices to assess a patient? Can it be used on its own?

BAKER: No it cannot; the scale is developed as a complementary measure to changes in seizure frequency, changes in the type of the seizures, changes in other parameters.

CRAMER: While the VA-scale has been used in research, Wijsman et al. used the scale in clinical practice. In order to validate their Composite Index of Impairment they used the concept that if a patient has more severe and more frequent seizures, you probably want to see him in the clinic more often. Indeed the correlation of the score with the frequency of visits had a good statistical outcome. In their score, similar to that in the VA composite score it is not just the number or the severity of the seizures, but also aspects of the treatment and the quantification of the adverse drug effects that form the score.

MARTINS DA SILVA: To return to the question of Dr. Keyser, I would like just to explain a little bit what we have done with the Chalfont centre seizure severity scale. It was not used to measure fluctuations of severity, but to control one of our variables. Severity was meant to be constant. We selected patients with a stable seizure severity in order to analyze the influence of frequency. One of our conclusions was that one cannot look at frequency without considering seizure type and seizure duration. Seizure duration, of course, especially if you are dealing with clusters of seizures, is related to frequency of seizures, because to define a frequency you need to have time in the denominator so the duration is an important characteristic of frequency. We encountered this problem in particular when we looked at brief seizures causing TCI (transient cognitive impairment). You really need to relate frequency with other parameters and to put them into one scale.

DUNCAN: One of the concerns I have about Dr. Martins da Silva's data is that he has Chalfont seizure severity scale scores going back to 1987, which is four years before the scale was invented. So I am concerned that a lot of his data has been derived from patient's records retrospectively, and I think that is probably an invalid procedure. I think this data has to be acquired at each clinic visit covering the time since the last visit, with the patient at least being prewarned prospectively about the factors that one is going to ask about, so as to get an accurate record.

KEYSER: What are the statistician's points of view on this topic?

JOHNSON: I want to raise one or two points. We have heard about the three scales developed in the U.S.A., Chalfont and Liverpool and the rating systems used in them. But so far there has been no mention of what is the basis upon which weights have been allocated. In particular I would like to know how the sensitivity of these scales would have changed, if other weighting factors had been applied. In addition to that, I would like to see how the total score on these scales relates to the individual items, in other words, whether any of those particular items, are actually predominantly driving or weighting the scale score.

I think that is particularly important as regards the issue of severity of seizures and frequency. We have no evidence at all as to the degree of association between the two.

I would like to make another point: it is sensible to try to keep the scale to measure severity of seizures simple. If we overload it with other complex issues such as serum concentrations there will be a trade-off between the different dimensions.

I am a little afraid if clinical trials would solely be evaluated by such scales. As a statistician I would have immense difficulty to determine the number of patients required to arrive at a clinically useful conclusion. I would first want to know the score difference which it is clinically important to detect and what is the variation in that. Only when we have information of that type, can we sit down and use the score in clinical trials.

CRAMER: I refer you to the VA study design that carefully evaluated the sample size based on estimation of clinically important differences in scale scores.

SPILKER: There is also the problem of missing data. Missing data are by far the most important problem for any clinical trial or epidemiological study. If we have missing data it is an awful problem to deal with in analysis. We cannot just throw out those patients with missing data and analyze those that have complete data, and expect to get unbiased estimates of treatment effects. If we take an alternative view and try to use some complex statistical modelling approach to actually substitute for missing data, that's fine for the statisticians but nobody else understands it and therefore they won't believe the results. Partly this is due to the fact that neither clinicians nor statisticians, just deep down, like the idea of creating data, whether it's done with a sophisticated model, simple averaging to get imputation, last observation carried forward, or anything else. And a major difficulty with rating scales is that you can have the most superb rating scale that you can devise—very high sensitivity, very high specificity, and fantastic positive predictive value—but if you cannot get the patients to come to your clinic to complete it, then it is totally useless. Actually missing data are not a problem for analysis; they are a problem for design and you should design your study in a way that minimizes the amount of missing data that you end up with. If you conduct a study which has a vast proportion of missing data, that is a reflection of poor study design and execution.

MEINARDI: Dr. Duncan what is the impact of your scale on patient management and what harm would missing data do? I mean, how much do you rely on this instrument?

DUNCAN: At the moment we do not rely at all on this instrument in routine clinical practice. It is premature. We are still going through the validation process. For example the people who have filled out the scales so far are people who have been involved in its development. What we are doing now is to turn the scale over to people who have no connection with the development of the scale, determining how reliable the data is, when obtained by personnel who have received minimum training in its use.

MEINARDI: What are your goals in the future for this scale?

DUNCAN: We would hope that the scale is a useful measure of anti-epileptic drug efficacy; further that it will provide useful objective data for inclusion in an Epilepsy Quality of Life scale and in assessments of patients' care requirements.

SPILKER: I have several questions about the validation of your scale. The first point is to choose the golden standard. People usually look at existing scales. I was wondering if you had any chance to compare your scale to other scales? You yourself listed three others. Did you see how the same patient rates using those scales? You really want a scale that is going to be sensitive to drug therapy. I think if you compare your scale with the other scales, and see how they did during drug treatment relative to treatment with another drug or relative to drug free patients, you would begin to see which scale is the most sensitive.

DUNCAN: We have considered all these points. Gus Baker and I have had a discussion over the last year about mutually using our seizure-severity scales, or to give them to a third party to see how they got along with them. The VA scale could be analyzed in the same way. With respect to drug effects the scales are being used in a double blind evaluation as part of a controlled study, but we do not yet have the results of this. One of the incentives to develop a scale was that patients were coming to the clinic saying "My seizures are not different in number but they are less severe" and we realize we are now getting a handle on that.

PORTER: The idea of comparing scale A with scale B with scale C might over time improve the reliability of the scale in terms of making sure you are measuring the same thing and having the same kind of data. But you do not convince me that this concept of sensibility proves the validity of the measures. Looking at Feinstein's paper the reason to abandon validation of sensitivity and validity is that the sum of measures cannot be validated. Yet the question I would ask is: "to what degree do we abandon the concept of validation of an index in the name of its sensitivity to the issues we want to measure?".

SPILKER: You are in a difficult position if there is no golden standard. I think the answer is: you make a start with your index, as people here around the table have made a start with their scales. If you are conducting a drug trial, you may get very accurate data with a scale, but perhaps the scale is not going to be responsive to drugs. Therefore, that scale would have to be rejected in a drug study at least. In terms of your question of face validity, if the measures assess what you really want them to, then that is good. In order to check if they are assessing correctly you have to use your best clinical judgment and then try to improve the quality of the assessment as you proceed. But that will be a very slow approach.

HEALTH STATUS IN EPILEPSY CARE

Aristides Kazis, M.D. and Sevasti Bostantjopoulou, M.D.

Aristotle University of Thessaloniki
3rd Department of Neurology
"G. Papanikolaou" Hospital
57010 Thessaloniki, Greece

Since the social implications of epilepsy are well known, the ultimate aim of treatment is to help the individual to achieve a satisfactory life adjustment. This can be done by complete control of seizures with no adverse effects. Although Rodin (1968) concluded that 80% of patients with epilepsy will not achieve seizure control, recent studies give a more optimistic picture with 58–82% of patients having a 2–5 year remission (Annegers et al 1979; Okuma and Kumashiro 1981; Elwes et al 1984). There remain a great number of patients needing specifically selected health services. According to many investigators epilepsy becomes chronic unless effectively treated at the onset. Reynolds (1989) reported that the first two years of treatment were critical in determining the future course and prognosis. Thus when dealing with a patient with epilepsy, in order to achieve complete control of seizures and consequently have a good prognosis, one must consider seizure type as well as other parameters, such as age at onset of epilepsy, sex, concomitant neurological or systemic diseases.

I. PATIENTS WITHOUT ANY OTHER HEALTH PROBLEMS EXCEPT EPILEPSY

Age and Epilepsy

Age and development influence factors governing excitability and inhibition, therefore they are important parameters of incidence rate.

Studies on experimental models of epilepsy have shown that the threshold for epileptic seizures is decreased in immature animals. The cortex of the premature and neonate is poorly organized for the propagation of seizures (Vining and Freeman 1986); therefore the immature brain is more susceptible than the mature brain to acute reactive seizures but it is difficult to sustain epileptic activity. The ability to fire and sustain firing

Quantitative Assessment in Epilepsy Care, Edited by H. Meinardi et al.
Plenum Press, New York, 1993

increases as the cortex matures. During childhood there is a period of time when, although the cortex becomes more capable of sustaining firing, the control mechanisms are not well developed thus explaining the increased incidence of epilepsy in children (Vining and Freeman 1986). As the cortex matures it develops control mechanisms to inhibit excessive discharges. Further studies have shown that the threshold for seizures is increased in aged animals. So the increase in the incidence of epilepsy in the elderly can be attributed to acquired or secondary epileptogenic disturbances.

When we are dealing with antiepileptic drugs in children we must have in mind that:

(1) Children metabolize drugs more quickly than adults so the dose/kg body weight should be higher than the adult and the half-life will be shorter and therefore the fluctuation in plasma levels will be greater (more frequent dosing compared with the adult) and

(2) The impact of medication on learning and behaviour is of great importance.

Experimental studies showed that young rats exposed to phenobarbital (PB) have decreased brain size and in cell cultures of cortical neurons PB and phenytoin (PHT) decreased choline acetyltransferase activity (Vining and Freeman 1986).

For neonates and infants PB is the drug of choice for a variety of seizures having the advantage of being available for parenteral administration. In children PB is associated with a high incidence of behavioral problems (such as sedation, hyperkinetic syndrome with overactivity, cognitive dysfunction, problems in memory and school performance). Phenytoin (PHT) is not the drug of choice for children because, apart from changes in cognitive function and behaviour, it is implicated in dysmorphic problems.

Carbamazepine (CBZ) is the drug of choice for children because it is relatively free of side effects as far as cognition and behaviour are concerned. Valproate (VPA) is implica ted in fatal hepatotoxicity in infants and children below the age of 2. Moreover these children on polytherapy have a one in 500 to 800 chance of developing fatal hepatotoxicity. Patients on negligible risk are those over the age of 10 on monotherapy while children between 2–10 years of age are at intermediate risk (Dreifuss et al. 1989).

Elderly patients may have diminished hepatic function (with respect to oxidative drug metabolism) and renal function and may require smaller doses of drugs. There is no difference among the first line anticonvulsant drugs although the diminished tendency of VPA and CBZ to produce cognitive impairment is important in this group of patients in whom there are already impairments due to cerebral disease. Anticonvulsant monitoring is useful in elderly patients especially when they are taking other drugs. The incidence of recurrence on withdrawal increases with age because there is usually a focal cerebral cause.

Pregnancy

The coexistence of pregnancy and epilepsy is a serious neurological problem. There are five subjects to deal with trying to solve this problem: effects of pregnancy on epilepsy, effects of epilepsy on pregnancy, effects of pregnancy on antiepileptic drug utilization, effects of epilepsy on the offspring and finally effects of antiepileptic drugs on the fetus, newborn and breast milk.

Effects of Pregnancy on Epilepsy

Although earlier studies showed that women with epilepsy experience an increase in seizure frequency, recent studies reported that seizure frequency remained unchanged in 58% of patients, increased in 28% and decreased in 14% (Saber and Dam 1990). Deterioration is seen in the first and third trimester. Reasons for increase in seizure frequency includes psychological factors and hormonal changes. The most reliable predictor of the course of epilepsy during pregnancy is the pregestational seizure frequency. Women who convulse at least once monthly before pregnancy usually worsen during pregnancy, while in women remaining seizure free for 9 months preceding pregnancy the risk of exacerbation is reduced to 20–40% (Donaldson 1986). Those who remained seizure free for the previous two years and/or have idiopathic generalized epilepsy are not likely to have seizure exacerbation during pregnancy. Status epilepticus is not more common in pregnant than in nonpregnant women. Although there is a great risk for mother and fetus, normal infants have been born thereafter (Saber and Dam 1990).

Effects of Epilepsy on Pregnancy

Older studies suggested reduced fertility in epileptic women but more recent studies have not found any reduction in fertility. Whether spontaneous abortion and toxaemia are more frequent in epileptic patients is controversial. Incidence of vaginal bleeding varies from 5.1% to 31% (controls 2.2–26%) (Saber and Dam 1990). There is a controversy whether incidence of vaginal bleeding increases during pregnancy in epileptic women. Moreover antiepileptic drugs increase the risk of folate deficiency during pregnancy.

Effects of Pregnancy on Monitoring Antiepileptic Drug Levels

Serum concentration levels of antiepileptic drugs fall during pregnancy. This is due to reduced gastric motility and secretion, increased hepatic metabolism and fall of the concentration of plasma proteins thus resulting in increased clearance and decreased total plasma concentration (Saber and Dam 1990).

Although the serum concentration of antiepileptic drugs is reduced, pharmacologically free fraction increases, so we have to measure blood levels each month in order to keep them at the lower limit of therapeutic range.

Effects of Seizures and of Antiepileptic Drugs on the Offspring and Newborn

Generalised convulsions with prolonged hypoxia and lactic acidosis are potentially dangerous for the fetus. Fetal heart rate decreases for more than 20 minutes after grand mal seizures but not after absences. Perinatal mortality rate is three times higher (Saber and Dam 1990).

Mental retardation, microcephaly, low birth weight and low Apgar scores occur with greater frequency in women with seizures. Hyperactivity, tremor, vomiting, irritability, poor weight gain and tachypnea may be seen in infants born to mothers taking barbiturates or diazepam (Saber and Dam 1990). Severe sedation with apnoea, cyanosis and hypotonia may be seen in neonates born to mothers treated with clonazepam. A bleeding tendency among newborns exposed to PHT and PB can be prevented by the administration of vitamin K during the last month of pregnancy.

There is little doubt that chronic antiepileptic drug treatment during the first trimester of pregnancy increases the risk of minor and major malformations in the child. The risk of congenital malformation, orofacial clefts, cardiac abnormalities and digital defects is increased two fold for offspring of treated epileptic women (2–4 times for facial cleft and 1–7 times for cardiac abnormalities) (Friis 1990). There is no substantial support for a common genetic predisposition between epilepsy and congenital malformations. Seizures during the first trimester of pregnancy are not considered as an important risk factor of inducing major congenital malformations.

Although enhanced teratogenic effects of PHT (fetal hydantoin syndrome) and PB have been reported, these claims have not been substantiated (Dalessio 1985). Polypharmacy and high drug levels increase the potential for problems during pregnancy. It is already known that there is 1–2% risk of neural tube defects in offsprings born to mothers treated with VPA (Editorial 1988; Friis 1990). Carbamazepine seems to be relatively safe with regard to risk of inducing major congenital malformations.

The concentration of antiepileptic drugs in fetal plasma is identical with maternal except for VPA which has higher fetal plasma levels. The amount of antiepileptic drug in the breast milk in negligible. Transmission rate of antiepileptic drug into the breast milk is 2% for VPA, 30% for PHT, 40% for PB and 45% for CBZ (Commission on Genetics, Pregnancy, and the Child, International League Against Epilepsy 1989).

Therefore every epileptic woman before getting pregnant should be informed about all these complications that may happen during pregnancy and delivery.

II. PATIENTS WITH SYMPTOMATIC EPILEPSY DUE TO NEUROLOGICAL DISORDER

Acquired brain lesions alter the anatomical pattern of epileptic susceptibility by lowering or raising seizure threshold in specific cerebral areas.

The pattern or type of seizures varies not only with the cause and location of the lesion but also with the degree of maturation of the brain.

It is said that symptomatic epilepsy is more difficult to treat than idiopathic epilepsy. However there is no thorough investigation about this subject.

Infections

Infections accounted for 3% of seizures in the Rochester study (Hauser and Kurland 1975). Meningitis, encephalitis, abscesses and granuloma induce active epileptic seizures but also residual structural change acts as a chronic epileptic lesion.

Annegers et al (1988) reported that the risk of developing late seizures after meningitis or encephalitis was 6.8%. The risk was 22% for patients with viral encephalitis and early seizures, 10% for patients with viral encephalitis without early seizures, 13% for patients with bacterial meningitis and early seizures, 2.4% for patients with bacterial meningitis without early seizures and 2.1% for patients with aseptic meningitis. Almost all investigators agree that epilepsy resulting from severe herpes simplex encephalitis is characterized by complex partial seizures which are intractable to treatment (Janz 1989). Furthermore patients who survive from an acute cerebral abscess develop seizures that are difficult to control with drugs (Legg et al 1973).

Neoplasms

Neoplasms accounted for 4% of seizures in the Rochester study (Hauser and Kurland 1975). Epileptic seizures occur in 20% to 70% of patients with intracranial tumours, especially of frontal, temporal and central areas and particularly with slowly growing ones. Gliomas are the most commonly encountered unsuspected neoplasm in surgical specimens (Engel 1989). These small lesions are associated with a long history of seizures.

The seizures are often partial in type. Thus, adult onset simple partial seizures which are refractory to drugs should alert the physician for the possibility of tumour. Chesterman et al (1987) found that three times more patients with structural lesions failed to achieve remission with a single drug. However a positive response to therapy does not rule out the possibility of tumour. On the other hand focal epilepsy with visible lesion should not be considered resistant to treatment per se.

Cerebral angioma causes epilepsy in about 40% of patients. The seizures are usually partial and may be difficult to treat (Shorvon 1986).

Cerebrovascular Disorders

Cerebrovascular disease is the most common etiology for epileptic seizures in older patients. However, studies on seizure related to stroke are relatively few and give controversial results.

Epileptic seizures are well recognised to occur both in the context of acute stroke (acute reactive seizures) in 10–15% of patients or as a sequel to it in 15% (Engel 1989).

Controversy exists whether epileptic seizures are more common in cerebral haemorrhage or infarction (Kilpatrick et al 1990; Black et al 1983). Shinton et al (1988) suggested that seizures were not particularly common in any pathological stroke sub-type.

The carotid area is implicated in the presence of epileptic seizures. There are no reports of patients with seizures in association with stroke in the area of the vertebral artery (Shinton et al 1988). Superficial cortical lesions are likely to cause seizures although there are reports with seizures in association with deep lesions (lacunas) (Olsen 1984; Shinton et al 1988; Kilpatrick et al 1990).

As far as intracerebral haemorrhage is concerned the location of the haematoma is important for the development of seizures. Lobar haematomas have the highest incidence of early, late and recurrent seizures (Berger et al 1988; Sung and Chu 1989).

Early seizures in acute stroke are usually simple partial. The indication for anticonvulsant drugs in patients with early seizures is controversial. Most studies described seizures to be readily controlled with drugs while other studies suggested that antiepileptic drugs are unhelpful because seizures usually resolve spontaneously. Seizures are not associated with higher mortality or worse functional outcome and do not predict the onset of a chronic recurrent epilepsy (Kilpatrick et al 1990).

The late development of partial and generalized seizures is due to glial scars sometimes associated with haemosiderin deposits. According to De Carolis et al (1984) late seizures are more common in middle cerebral artery occlusive disease because of higher risk of haemorrhage in the cortical infarct. It has been suggested that the risk of recurrent seizures is higher in patients with late seizures (Lesser et al 1985). Gupta et al (1988) reported recurrent seizures in 30% of patients with both early and late seizures.

Furthermore silent infarctions have an increased prevalence in patients with late onset epilepsy (Roberts et al 1988). So cerebrovascular disease is probably the major underlying contributing factor for the development of epilepsy in older patients without other apparent etiologic diagnosis and, generally speaking, the seizures in cerebrovascular epilepsy are relatively responsive to treatment.

Post-traumatic Epilepsy

Post-traumatic seizures are divided, on the basis of the latency period between trauma and first seizure in early and late onset seizures.

Early post traumatic seizures, that is seizures occurring within 5 min to 1 week after trauma, occur in about 1.9–5% of all patients with head injury (Annegers et al 1980; Janz 1989). They occur more frequently in children (4–12%) even after minor head trauma (Majkowski 1990).

In about 25–30% of the cases they occur during the first hour after head injury with a highest prevalence in the first week and then there is a sharp decline (Majkowski 1990).

Early seizures are usually partial in type. They are the expression of a direct effect of trauma. Although they seem to indicate the presence of severe concussion they tend to cease spontaneously.

There are many risk factors predisposing to early epileptic seizures. Especially the length of unconsciousness or the post traumatic amnesia play an important role (Janz 1989; Majkowski 1990).

The average risk of early seizures to persist is about 25%. It increases to 45% in the case of open injuries, lies between 13–27% in the case of medium and severe closed injuries and drops to 0% in the case of mild head trauma (Annegers et al 1980; Janz 1989).

The occurrence of the first late seizure is more than 7 days after head trauma. The upper range of latency may be 10–15 or even 20 years. In about 95% of cases first late seizure occur within the first 3 years after head trauma.

According to the majority of authors the risk of late seizures (which are mainly partial complex) varies for all kinds of closed injuries from 2% to about 6% (Majkowski 1990). The risk increases to about 36–53% in cases of war injuries with penetration of dura (the risk is greater, about 70%, when wound infections occur), to 35% in the case of intracranial haematoma and up to 17% in the case of depressed fracture (Salazar et al

1985; Janz 1989). The risk is greater when the lesion is close to the central sulcus. The prognosis of late seizures is not necessarily unfavourable so that epilepsy does not develop in all cases.

A number of studies of prophylactic treatment have been published using a variety of drugs (CBZ, VPA, PHT) with controversial results. The questions as to which drug in which dosage and how long treatment should last have not been answered yet. Janz (1989) suggested that the attempt to prevent early seizures with drugs in not indicated. Most authors propose to start AED after a first seizure or until two seizures occurred in a brief interval. Early reactive seizures are not an indication for continued treatment after 1 year. Prophylactic treatment for early seizures with high plasma concentrations of phenytoin when there is a great risk for early repeated seizures or status (children under the age of 5, intracranial haematoma) might be reasonable. PHT has been reported to prevent the development of chronic seizures following experimental focal neocortical lesions induced by alumina in the cat while PB and CBZ exert a prophylactic effect on amygdaloid kindling in the cat (Engel 1989).

Although experimental and uncontrolled clinical trials suggest that prophylactic AED reduces the incidence of traumatic late seizures a large controlled study has indicated no such effect (Young et al 1985).

Since there is a controversy about the duration of treatment most investigators propose a gradual discontinuation after 1 year if no seizures occur after the acute post traumatic period.

Furthermore we must have in mind an important phenomenon demonstrated in animal study—the "conditioned inefficacy." This data suggests that inadequate prophylaxis may be worse than no prophylaxis (Engel 1989).

So even with the higher risk of epilepsy the usefulness and risks of treatment should be assesses with the patient.

III. PATIENTS WITH EPILEPSY AND SYSTEMIC DISORDERS

Hepatic Failure

In hepatic failure there is a reduction of drug metabolizing activity and disruption of hepatic vascular architecture causing inhibition of drug metabolism and prolongation of half lives (Richens 1986; Perucca and Richens 1989; Johannessen et al 1990). Furthermore lower albumin levels result in a decrease in the extent of binding of the high-protein bound drugs and an increase in free fraction in plasma. So blood AED levels must be frequently monitored and the dose must be adjusted carefully.

Only serious hepatic failure influences drug metabolism therefore there is no reason for changing the medication (except withdrawal of valproate).

Diazepam is the drug of choice but with smaller doses and longer dosage interval. Paraldehyde may be given because it is eliminated by the lungs.

Renal Failure

Excretion of drugs and their metabolites is reduced in renal failure so there is a risk of accumulation and intoxication. Furthermore there are changes in the protein binding, distribution and metabolism (Richens 1986; Perucca and Richens 1989). Therefore in patients with impaired renal function the dosage of drugs which are excreted unchanged must be individualized on the basis of the glomerular filtration rate.

Again diazepam is the drug of choice. Phenytoin may be used but we must have in mind the protein binding capacity for phenytoin is reduced so there is an increased free fraction and the elimination rate is increased. Paraldehyde also can be used.

Cardiovascular Diseases

In patients with congestive heart failure CBZ can cause water retention and should not be used (Engel 1989).

Seizures due to rheumatic heart diseases or cardiac arrythmia are relatively responsive to treatment.

Gastrointestinal Disorders

There is a potential for disturbed drug absorption in patients with severe gastrointestinal disease therefore we should always monitor the plasma levels of the drugs.

Porphyria

Seizures occasionally occur with acute porphyria and create a particular problem because AED exacerbate the porphyric state.

Diazepam and paraldehyde are safe for the treatment of status epilepticus and clonazepam is an alternative (Engel 1989).

For chronic treatment bromide is the only entirely safe medication (Engel 1989).

IV. PATIENTS WITH EPILEPSY ON DRUGS FOR VARIOUS DISEASES

The use of multiple drugs has created the problem of drug interaction which can cause various side effects, even life threatening ones.

Drug interactions can occur at many levels, however many of them are due to modification in absorption, distribution, biotransformation or excretion (Plaa 1989). However, the mechanism of other drug interactions is not well understood.

Drugs more prone to result in interactions are those whose pharmacologic actions are affected by modification in plasma concentration. Dangerous drugs interactions are those involving the combination of different drugs that affect the pharmacokinetics of coumarin type anticoagulants, oral hypoglycaemic agents and agents acting on the myocardium.

Patients on Anticoagulant Drugs

Phenytoin reduces the blood level of dicoumarol resulting in a need for increased dosage of dicoumarol. The effect of phenytoin on warfarin is variable (Kutt 1989).

Bishydroxycoumarin causes elevation of plasma phenytoin levels in some patients.

Carbamazepine decreases action of warfarin. Finally dicoumarol action is increased by valproate.

Patients on Cardiac Drugs

Amiodarone causes an increase of plasma phenytoin levels. Phenytoin reduces the half life of quinidine by 50% and make it necessary to administer larger doses of quinidine (Kutt 1989). In addition phenytoin reduces digitoxin levels. Verapamil and diltiazem double CBZ concentrations.

Carbamazepine

Calcium channel blockers have variable effects on CBZ metabolism. Verapamil and diltiazem double CBZ concentrations but not nifedipine (Pitlick and Levy 1989). Cimetidine increases CBZ concentration but this interaction is of modest clinical significance.

Erythromycin causes CBZ intoxication (drowsiness, nausea, vomiting). The same happens with triacetyloleandomycin and propoxyphene. Furthermore CBZ decreases action of theophylline and oral contraceptives (Engel 1989).

Valproate

Salicylic acid displaces VPA from protein, resulting in higher free VPA levels. In addition aspirin changes VPA metabolism by competing with VPA for mitochondrial oxidation (Mattson and Cramer 1989).

Phenytoin

Salicylates displace phenytoin from the plasma protein binding sites, causing an increase of the unbound fraction from 10% to 16% (Kutt 1989). Cimetidine inhibits phenytoin metabolism increasing plasma concentrations. Phenytoin induces metabolism of dexamethasone and oral contraceptives, and increases the rate of clearance of theophylline.

In conclusion, epilepsy is not a simple subject to deal with. Other elements apart from seizure frequency and severity should be also taken into account when treating epileptic patients.

Health status of such patients should be considered as a whole in order to achieve the maximum results in epilepsy care efforts, either in prophylaxis or in seizure treatment itself.

REFERENCES

Annegers JF. Hauser WA. Elveback LR. Remission of seizures and relapse in patients with epilepsy. Epilepsia 1979; 20: 729–737.

Annegers JF. Grabow JD. Groover RV et al. Seizures after head trauma: a population study. Neurology 1980; 30: 683–689.

Annegers JF. Hauser WA. Beghi E et al. The risk of unprovoked seizures after encephalitis and meningitis. Neurology 1988; 38: 1407–1410.

Berger AR. Lipton RB. Lesser ML et al. Early seizures following intracerebral hemorrhage: implications for therapy. Neurology 1988; 38: 1363–1365.

Black SE. Norris JW. Hachinski VC. Post-stroke seizures. Stroke 1983; 14: 134.

Chesterman P. Elwes RDC. Reynolds EH. Failure of monotherapy in newly diagnosed epilepsy. In: Wolf P. Dam M. Janz D. Dreifuss E. eds. Advances in epileptology: XVIth Epilepsy International Symposium New York: Raven Press, 1987: 461–464.

Commission on Genetics, Pregnancy, and the Child, International League Against Epilepsy. Guidelines for the Care of epileptic women of childbearing age. Epilepsia 1989; 30: 409–410.

Dalessio DJ. Current concepts: Seizure disorders and pregnancy. N Engl J Med 1985; 312: 559–563.

De Carolis P. D'Alessandro R. Ferrara R et al. Late seizures in patients with internal carotid and middle cerebral artery occlusive disease following ischaemic events. J Neurol Neurosurg Psychiatry 1984; 47: 1345–1347.

Donaldson JO. Neurologic complications of pregnancy. In: Asbury AK. McKhann GM. McDonald WI eds. Diseases of the nervous system. Philadelphia: WB. Saunders Company 1986: 1578–1584.

Dreifuss FE. Langer DH. Moline KA. and Maxwell JE. Valproic acid hepatic fatalities. II US experience since 1984. Neurology 1989; 39: 201–207.

Editorial. Valproate, spina bifida, and birth defect registries. Lancet 1988; ii: 1404–1405.

Elwes RDC. Johnson AL. Shorvon SD. Reynolds EH. The prognosis for seizure control in newly diagnosed epilepsy. N Engl J Med 1984; 311: 944–947.

Engel J. ed. Seizures and epilepsy Philadelphia: F.A. Davis Company 1989.

Friis ML. Malformations in children of epileptic patients. In: Dam M. Gram L. eds. Comprehensive Epileptology. New York: Raven Press 1990: 309–319.

Gupta SR. Naheedy MH, Elias D. Rubino FA. Postinfarction seizures: a clinical study. Stroke 1988, 19: 1477–1481.

Hauser WA. Kurland LT. The epidemiology of epilepsy in Rochester, Minnesota, 1935 through 1967. Epilepsia 1975; 16: 1–66.

Janz D. Prognosis and prophylaxis of traumatic epilepsy. In: Trimble MR. ed. Chronic epilepsy, its prognosis and management. Chichester: John Wiley and sons 1989: 87–102.

Janz D. How does one assess the severity of epilepsy? In: Trimble MR. ed. Chronic epilepsy, its prognosis and management. Chichester: John Wiley & sons 1989: 21–36.

Johannessen SI. Loyning V. Munthekaas AW. General aspects. In: Dam M. Gram L. eds. Comprehensive Epileptology. New York: Raven Press 1990; 505–524.

Kutt H. Phenytoin. Interactions with other drugs. In: Levy R. Mattson R. Meldrum B. et al. eds. Antiepileptic Drugs, Third Edition. New York: Raven Press 1989: 215–232.

Legg NJ. Gupta PC. Scott DF. Epilepsy following cerebral abscess: a clinical and EEG study of 70 patients. Brain 1973; 96: 259–268.

Lesser RP. Luders H. Dinner DS. Morris HH. Epileptic seizures due to thrombotic and embolic cerebro-vascular disease in older patients. Epilepsia 1985; 26: 622–630.

Majkowski J. Posttraumatic epilepsy. In: Dam M. Gram L. eds. Comprehensive Epileptology. New York: Raven Press 1990: 281–298.

Mattson RH. Cramer JA. Valproate interactions with other drugs. In: Levy R. Mattson R. Meldrum B. et al. eds. Antiepileptic Drugs, Third edition. New York: Raven Press 1989; 621–632.

Okuma T. Kumashiro H. Natural history and prognosis of epilepsy: report of a multi-institutional study in Japan. Epilepsia 1981; 22: 35–53.

Olsen TS. Factors of importance for the development of epilepsy in patients with cerebral infarction. Acta Neurol Scand 1984; 69 (suppl) 95–96.

Perucca E. Richens A. General Principles. Biotransformation. In: Levy R. Mattson R. Meldrum B. et al eds. Antiepileptic Drugs, Third Edition. New York: Raven Press, 1989: 23–48.

Pitlick WH. Levy RH. Carbamazepine: Interactions with other drugs. In: Levy R. Mattson R. Meldrum B. et al. eds. Antiepileptic Drugs, Third Edition. New York: Raven Press, 1989: 521–531.

Plaa GL. General Principles. Toxicology. In: Levy R. Mattson R. Meldrum B. et al. eds. Antiepileptic Drugs, Third Edition: New York: Raven Press, 1989: 49–58.

Reynolds EH. The prognosis of epilepsy: is chronic epilepsy preventable? In: Trimble MR. ed. Chronic epilepsy, its prognosis and management. Chichester: John Wiley and Sons 1989: 13–20.

Richens A. Anticonvulsant pharmacokinetics. In: Asbury AK, McKhann GM. McDonald WI. eds. Diseases of the nervous system. Philadelphia: WB. Saunders Company 1986: 1001–1007.

Roberts RC. Shorvon SD. Cox TCS. Gilliatt RW. Clinically unsuspected cerebral infarction revealed by computed tomography scanning in late onset epilepsy. Epilepsia 1988; 29: 190–194.

Rodin EA. ed. The prognosis of patients with epilepsy. Springfield, IL: Thomas, 1968.

Saber A. Dam M. Pregnancy, delivery and puerperium. In: Dam M. Gram L. eds. Comprehensive Epileptology. New York: Raven Press 1990: 299–307.

Shinton RA. Gill JS. Melnich SC. et al. The frequency, characteristics and prognosis of epileptic seizures at the onset of stroke. J Neurol Neurosurg Psychiatry 1988; 51: 273– 276.

Shorvon SD. Classification of epilepsy. In: Asbury AK. McKhann GM. McDonald WI. eds. Diseases of the nervous system. Philadelphia: WB Saunders Company 1986; 970–981.

Sung CY. Chu NS. Epileptic seizures in intracerebral haemorrhage. J Neurol Neurosurg Psychiatry 1989; 52: 1273–1276.

Vining EPB, Freeman JM. Management of childhood seizures. In: Asbury AK. McKhann GM. McDonald WI. eds. Diseases of the nervous system. Philadelphia: WB. Saunders Company 1986; 1018–1032.

Young B. Rapp PR. Norton JA. et al. Failure of prophylactically administered phenytoin to prevent late post traumatic seizures. J Neurosurg 1983; 58: 231–235.

HEALTH STATUS IN EPILEPSY CARE: CLINIMETRIC APPROACH

P. Jallon, M.D.

Privat-Dozent
Chief, EEG Department
Hôpital Cantonal Universitaire de Genève
Genève, Switzerland

INTRODUCTION

Clinimetrics is "the science of quantification of clinical phenomena with particular attention to the validation of the outcome variables" (20). With such a definition, clinimetrics will be useful in the appreciation of the results of epidemiologic studies and the evaluation of the efficiency of drug therapy in clinical practice. (10)

The application of clinimetrics to epilepspy by the Veterans Administration Group has permitted the use of a *Composite Score* designed "to reflect the total effect of seizures and toxicity from medication on the quality of the patient's life" (7). Wijsman (20) has proposed a *Composite Index of Impairment* that "is constructed by correcting the index of seizure value and adding factors concerning impairment caused by side-effects of a treatment." The toxicity of a treatment can be assessed by evaluation of the VA systemic toxicity rating and the VA neurotoxicity rating.

Patients with epilepsy are not immune to the common diseases that affect the general population. The frequency of seizures and the response to antiepileptic drugs could differ markedly because of a medical disorder. Health status of epileptic patients may interfere with the evolution of the illness, and the therapeutic management of epilepsy. Health status can modify some parameters and must be taken into account into the quantification of phenomena and in the weighting of indices such as the seizure rating or the composite index of impairment. (fig.1)

In this paper, we would like to present some situations that can interfere with the weighting or the adjustment of indices proposed by Cramer and Wijsman, in the diagnosis, management, the therapeutic follow-up and the evaluation of the prognosis of epilepsy.

Quantitative Assessment in Epilepsy Care, Edited by H. Meinardi et al.
Plenum Press, New York, 1993

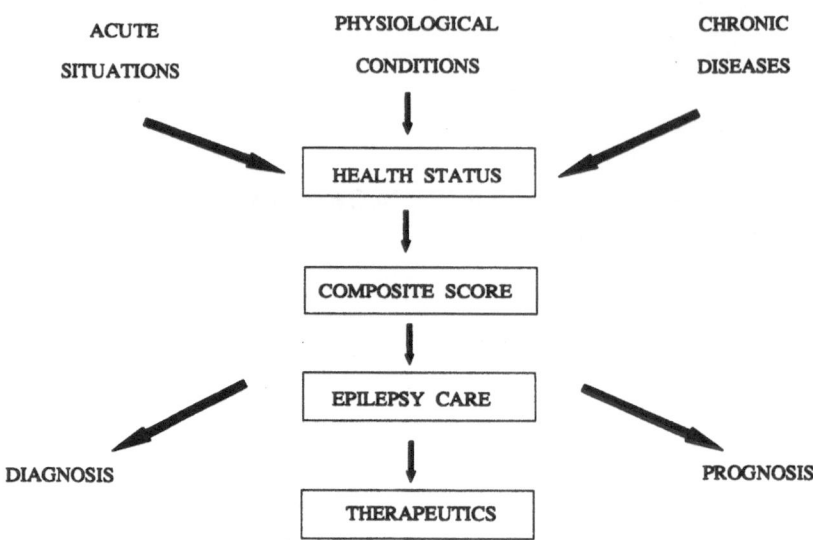

Figure 1. The role of health status in epilepsy care.

A. CLINIMETRIC INDICES

Indices that we are going to use in our discussion are adopted from the Veterans Administration rating scales.

Index of Seizures

"The seizure frequency rating grades each type of seizure based on frequency and severity of the seizure episodes." (7) This rating score is divided into three sections following semiology of the seizures: (1) generalized tonic-clonic seizures, (2) complex partial seizures, (3) simple partial seizures. We agree with Cramer et al. (7) that according to the index of severity, two generalized tonic-clonic seizures per year are equal to four complex partial seizures in a week or daily simple partial seizure. This seizure index is modulated by adding factors such as conscious first symptoms, nocturnal distribution of seizures, precipitating factors, and patient's compliance. Other seizure severity scales have been presented with a high degree of reliability and validity by Duncan and Sander from Chalfont Centre (8) and by Baker (4)

Index of Systemic Toxicity

This index is used "to quantify impairment or change in physical status that could occur with the use of antiepileptic drugs." (7) It is important to note in that quantification if the patient has long-standing problems before entering the study. In this case, only increased problems will be scored.

Index of Neurotoxicity

It is based on the evaluation of motor and sensory signs, cognitive function, level of sedation, affect and mood changes. The behavioral toxicity battery can be used to more closely determine changes in motor integrative functions, cognitive and memory functions and profiles of mood states.

The Composite Score

This index represents "the summation of the scores from the seizure rating, systemic toxicity rating and neurotoxicity rating combined with the behavioral toxicity rating" (7). This composite score is completed during an initial visit and evaluated at every follow up visit by the physician.

B. HEALTH STATUS

The rating scores that we have adopted could be modified or modulated by different situations that must be integrated in baseline data.

Three types of situations could be examined:

(1) **Acute situations** can modify rating score during a short time.

- Children, most often or adults receiving carbamazepine and macrolide antibiotic therapy (troleandomycin, erythromycin, josamycin) can produce acute systemic intoxication symptoms and neurotoxicity signs after three to seven days of co-administration.

- Acute psychiatric disturbances can interfere with the neurotoxicity index because the use of psychotropic drugs in association with antiepileptic drugs such as phenothiazines and phenytoin.

- An acute alcoholic intoxication increases the risk of multiple and severe seizures by a withdrawal mechanism or in a metabolic way such as an hypoglycaemia.

All these situations are brief, transient episodes that can lead to a change in drug regimen or can interfere as a modifier of seizure severity scale.

(2) Some **situations, without being pathological,** could interfere in the evolution of epileptic illness and can modify rating of the composite index.

(2.1) Pregnancy.   In itself, pregnancy does not cause epileptic seizures but numerous studies have shown that the course of epilepsy can change for the better or the worse during pregnancy. Janz et al. (13) have written that in about a quarter of women who had seizures before becoming pregnant, seizure frequency increases during pregnancy. In another quarter, frequency decreases, and in about half of the

cases, there is no change. Possible causes can explain the increase of seizure frequency during pregnancy: hormonal changes, metabolic factors, pharmacokinetic activations, or even psychological problems.

So, can pregnancy modify seizure index? The variation in seizure frequency in the group of pregnant women should not modify the rating score of the seizure index. Conversely, pregnancy can interfere with the systemic toxicity index or neurotoxicity index because the consequences of an acute or a chronic intoxication by antiepileptic drugs are more harmful in a pregnant woman.

We think that in these cases, we could assign a weighted score.

(2.2) The Elderly. Numerous studies (e.g., Loiseau, 14) have shown that incidence of epileptic seizures increases in a striking way in elderly patients. The main reason for so high an incidence is the number of acute symptomatic seizures and situation related seizures. In addition to this group of patients with new onset of epilepsy, there will be a number of chronic epileptic patients who will have survived.

The pharmacodynamic differences between the elderly and younger people need to be considered: the elderly are more sensitive to the effects of drugs producing sedation and alteration of cognitive functions, especially with benzodiazepines. Pharmacokinetics parameters can influence serum levels (18): alteration of absorption, changes in binding to proteins, decreasing of the enzyme mass, reduction of the hepatic blood flow. Drug interactions represent a major problem in the therapy of epilepsy in the elderly, especially between cardioactive drugs and some of the anticonvulsants.

All these specific aspects can interfere with composite scores and particularly with the systemic rating score and neurotoxicity scores.

(3) **Some chronic diseases,** pathological states or organic dysfunction are going to interfere in the therapeutic management and with the consequences of the severity of the seizures.

(3.1) Major Organ Diseases. Patients with liver or kidney diseases often have adverse reactions to drugs, this is not surprising because these organs are involved in their elimination. Seizures are a frequent complication in patients with uraemia and are often associated with hepatic insufficiency. The use of antiepileptic drugs in association with a hepatic or kidney disease is far from uncommon.

- Antiepileptic drug metabolism occurs almost exclusively in the liver. Severe liver damage such as cirrhosis or a chronic active hepatitis can lead to significant prolongation of the half life of a drug, resulting in clinical toxicity.

- Renal diseases can significantly affect the disposition of antiepileptic drugs: it can impair urinary excretion of the drug or its metabolites; it can also affect the kinetics by altering protein binding, distribution or metabolism.

So if we apply these findings in a clinimetric approach, we could say that major organ diseases can affect seizure ratings because it will be difficult to establish adequate treatment and the risk of seizure recurrence is really increased.

The risk of systemic toxicity and neurotoxicity is high and we must assess a weighting rate to the composite score in case of renal or hepatic failures.

(3.2) Cardiac Diseases. Annegers (2) wrote the following in the conclusion of his paper about heart diseases and epilepsy: "Persons with epilepsy have a twofold increase of all causes of mortality: death rate for heart diseases are not increased overall in persons with epilepsy although there is a significant increase in patients under 65 years of age. The incidence of myocardial infarction is increased in patients with both idiopathic or remote symptomatic epilepsy." Satischandra (16) found a positive association between epilepsy and myocardial ischemia (odds ratio: 1.8).

Curiously, the association of cardiac diseases and epilepsy is not so frequently reported but we could imagine that the risk of sudden death is greatly increased in patients with cardiac arrhythmia, myocardial heart diseases or cardiac insufficiency.

The difficulty could be increased in case of use of phenytoin and carbamazepine for which the cardiac side effects are well known (9). We think that cardiac diseases could interfere with the composite impairment index in two ways, influencing the:

- seizure index, because consequences of frequency and severity of seizures are more important in an epileptic person with heart disease. (17, 19)

- systemic toxicity because drug interactions between cardiac drugs and antiepileptic drugs could be life threatening.

(3.3) Alcoholism. Some clinical studies have correlated alcohol abuse with poor seizure control (11). Patients with epilepsy must be warned of alcohol's potential for exacerbating seizures and be advised not to drink in excess. Numerous mechanisms could be suggested to explain the increase of the frequency of seizures in epileptic patients who consume alcohol: withdrawal effects, modification of antiepileptic drugs metabolism through hepatic induction, hypoglycaemia, non compliance. But the increase in seizure frequency occurs in individuals who drink frequently and heavily.

Alcoholism could interfere with the seizure index because risks of increasing the frequency of seizures and the risk of more frequent generalization. Alcoholism can increase the neurotoxicity index because the sites of neurotoxicity are the same for alcohol and antiepileptic drugs.

The difficulty is to weight the different scores and overall to assess the notion of alcoholism. Are there: clinical signs of chronic alcoholism ? biological signs of alcoholism? Is there a history of frequent drinking? Are the consequences of heavy drinking visible?

(3.4) Psychiatric Disturbances. It is obvious that there is a relationship between epilepsy and some psychiatric diseases, such as depression. Currie et al. (6) diagnosed depression in 11% of the patients with temporal lobe epilepsy in a British hospital based study.

The association of psychotropic drugs with antiepileptic drugs needs some precautions because many of these drugs lower the seizure threshold and can increase the frequency of seizures.

The association with severe psychiatric illness can interfere in rating scores such as the seizure severity index and the neurotoxicity index.

(3.5) Infectious Disease. Any infectious disease, by provoking fever, may increase the risk of a seizure. On the other hand, data from Rochester (1) have provided an increased risk of developing epilepsy among subjects who have encephalitis, which is slightly lower in case of meningitis.

The association of seizure and HIV infection has been stressed. The association would be evaluated to about 10 to 13%. (5) Status epilepticus and poorly controlled seizure are frequent. Holtzmann (12) had stressed that hypersensitivity reactions occurred in about 15% of patients treated with Phenytoin. This situation represents a good example of impact on the index of systemic toxicity.

CONCLUSIONS

It is clear that, from a medical point of view, health status is important to consider if we want to propose indexes of assessment of epilepsy. The difficulty is to select and/or to weigh attributes to develop scales.

Prospective and retrospective studies have to be made to develop rigorous scales based on "normal" situations. The modulation of scores by qualifiers in pathological situations could be made at a later stage. The use of indices indicating the severity of epilepsy in this population (epilepsy and abnormal health status) have to be tested for clinical applicability and validity.

REFERENCES

1. Annegers J.F, Hauser W.A, Beghi E. et al. The risk of unprovoked seizures after encephalitis and meningitis. Neurology 1988; 38: 1407–1410.
2. Annegers J.F, Hauser W.A, Shirts S.B. Heart Disease Mortality and Morbidity in Patients with Epilepsy.Epilepsia 1984; 25:699–704.
3. Asconapé J.J, Penry J.K. Use of Antiepileptic Drugs in the Presence of Liver and Kidney diseases: A Review. Epilepsia 1982; 23:S65–S79.
4. Baker G.B, Smith D.F, Dewey M., Morrow J., Crawford P.M, Chadwick D.W. The development of a seizure scale as an outcome measure in epilepsy. Epilepsy Res. 1991; 8:245–251.
5. Bartolomei F., Pellegrino P., Dhiver C., Quilichini R, Gastaut J.A, Gastaut J.L. Crises d'épilepsie au cours de l'infection par le VIH. La Presse Médicale 1991; 20:2135–2138.
6. Currie S., Heathfield KWG, Hewson R.A et al. Clinical course and prognosis of temporal lobe epilepsy.Brain 1971; 94: 173–190.
7. Cramer J.A, Smith D.B, Mattson R.H, Delgado-Escueta A.V, Collins J.F, and the V A Epilepsy Cooperative Study Group. A method of quantification for the evaluation of antiepileptic drug therapy. Neurology 1983; 33:26–37.
8. Duncan J.S, Sander J.W.A.S. The Chalfont Seizure Severity Scale. Journal of Neurology, Neurosurgery and Psychiatry 1991; 54873–876.
9. Durelli L, Mutani R., Sechi G.P, Monaco F.,Glorioso N., Gusmaroli G. Cardiac side effects of Phenytoin and Carbamazepine. Arch Neurol 1985; 42:1067–1068.
10. Feinstein A.R. Clinimetrics. New Haven:Yale University Press,1987.

11. Hauser W.A, Ng S.K.C, Brust J.C.M. Alcohol, Seizures and Epilepsy. Epilepsia,1988; 29: S66–S78.

12. Holtzman D.M, Kaku D.A, So Y.T. New-onset seizures associated with human immunodeficiency virus infection: Causation and clinical features in 100 cases.A.J.M.1989; 87:173–177.

13. Janz D. Antiepileptic drugs and pregnancy: altered utilization patterns and teratogenesis. Epilepsia 1982; 23: S53–S63.

14. Loiseau J, Loiseau P, Duché B, Guyot M, Dartigues J.F, Aublet B. A survey of epileptic disorders in Southwest France: Seizures in Elderly patients.Ann.Neurol:1990:27:232–237.

15. Reynolds E.H, Trimble M.R. Epilepsy and Psychiatry. Churchill Livingstone (1981) 279 pages

16. Satishchandra P, Chandra V, Schoenberg B.S. Case-Control Study of Associated Conditions at the Time of Death in Patients with Epilepsy. Neuroepidemiology 1988; 7:109–114.

17. Sechi G, Dessi-Fulgheri P, Glorioso N, Volta G, Rosati G. Myocardial Infarction Complicating Status Epilepticus. Epilepsia 1985; 26:572–576.

18. Troupin A.S, Johannessen S.I. Epilepsy in the Elderly. A Pharmacologic Perspective. In Epilepsy. Current Approaches to Diagnosis and Treatment. Smith D.B. edit. Raven Press 1990; 141–154.

19. Vesterby A, Gregersen M, Baandrup U. The Myocardium in Epileptics. The American Journal of Forensic Medecine and Pathology 1986; 7:288–290.

20. Wijsman D.J.P, Hekster Y.A, Keyser A, Renier W.O. Meinardi H. Clinimetrics and epilepsy care. Pharmaceutisch Weekblad Scientific edition 1991; 13:182–188.

DRUG CHOICE AND REPLACEMENT

D.G.A. Kasteleijn-Nolst Trenité, M.D.

Chief, Research Support Unit
Instituut voor Epilepsiebestrijding "Meer en Bosch"/"De Cruquiushoeve"
Achterweg 5
2103 SW Heemstede
The Netherlands

INTRODUCTION

In western society the great majority of patients suffering from epilepsy will receive drug treatment. The antiepileptic drugs (AEDs) will usually be prescribed for at least two or three years. The strategy and practice of AEDs description will be discussed with respect to two situations i.e. clinical practice and the search for better AEDs.

CLINICAL PRACTICE

For the individual patient different questions have to be answered in clinical practice. The first question is whether or not a patient should be treated with AEDs. There are various reasons for withholding drug treatment: uncertainty about the diagnosis of epilepsy, low seizure frequency or severity, a clear and consistent precipitation of seizures by a preventable action and the wish to get pregnant. Furthermore, the patient himself or his/her parents could be very reluctant to take medication on a regular daily base. Once the decision of drug treatment has been made, the question arises which drug and in what dosage this should be prescribed.

In routine clinical practice the choice of drug will be made by considering various aspects, such as type of seizures and/or epilepsy classification. This choice will also be dependent on age and sex of the patient, e.g. no treatment with phenytoin in female patients, and whether the patient has a history of allergic reactions (less likelihood of choosing carbamazepine or phenytoin). Also the level of intelligence and/or profession will generally be taken into account.

Quantitative Assessment in Epilepsy Care, Edited by H. Meinardi et al.
Plenum Press, New York, 1993

Besides parameters derived from the history of a patient, knowledge of the prescribing clinician him/herself will determine the drug choice. The knowledge of a clinician concerning pharmacokinetic and pharmacodynamic features of the various AEDs will have its influence on decision making. His/her apprehension depends on education (books, literature, teachers and other colleagues, pharmaceutical industry) and experience. Variability in these parameters can account for the observed differences in drug prescription by clinicians. In general, experience with prescription of AEDs has advantages, but can also prevent the clinician from changing his/her opinion.

The history of a patient in combination with knowledge of the doctor will finally lead to prescription of a certain amount of drug A (first choice). Nevertheless differences in choice of the drug, dosage, vehiculum and regimen, may be different between clinicians in various countries and even between clinicians in the same tertiary referral hospital for epileptic patients. Indeed, it is more likely that the prescription of AEDs is more uniform in the case of the clinician without much knowledge about epilepsy treatment.

Chronic Treatment

Generally, the patient will take the prescribed amount of drug A for approximately one to three months before evaluation of the effect on the seizures. The evaluation is dependent on the history of the patient concerning seizure frequency and severity, side-effects and allergic reactions. Most clinicians will also ask for laboratory tests: biochemical and haematological examinations and determination of the serum level of the prescribed AED. If a patient has complaints, clinical examination with emphasis on specific toxic signs will also be performed. Often a control EEG will be registered. The results of these investigations combined with the patient's history will lead to the decision to continue drug therapy with or without dose adaptation, change in formulation or regimen (individualization). Only when a patient has shown allergic reactions to the drug (fever, dermatological reaction, increase of fits), this drug will be withdrawn. In the majority of patients dose adaptation will be needed.

Even after considering non-compliance, about 30% of the patients will continue to have fits with the maximal dosage of the drug of first choice (Reynolds and Shorvon, 1981). A second AED will then be introduced as add-on therapy. Ideally, the first drug should be withdrawn whether or not the patient becomes seizure-free. However, in clinical practice it is general use not to change "a winning horse." Moreover, the patient him/herself often decides to continue the polytherapy in fear of relapse of seizures and consequent loss of driving licence, etc. In not-seizure-free patients, the search for a good combination of AEDs will continue and can last for many years.

Preferably any drug should be tried out in monotherapy, beginning with a low dosage and gradually increasing up to appearance of toxic signs and symptoms. However, if monotherapy fails to control seizures adequately, any combination of two drugs should be tried out. Again the type of seizures and/or epilepsy classification, age and sex, level of intelligence and profession etc. have to be taken into account in the choice of the additional drugs. Knowledge about the individual pharmacokinetic and dynamic reactions on already prescribed drugs will increase and has to play a role when choosing another type of AEDs.

In general, however, evaluation of the efficacy of a specific drug, given in polytherapy is difficult because of drug-drug interactions. Prescription of more then one drug at a time can complicate matters (Eadie and Tyrer, 1989). Every AED has its own pharmacokinetic and pharmacodynamic identity. There will be competition between the different drugs at levels of absorption, bio-availability, metabolism, amount of free fraction and clearance. Yet too little is known of pharmacokinetic and specific pharmacodynamic interactions between drugs to guide prescription of polytherapy. Even if some pharmacokinetic changes are known, e.g. increase in metabolism due to enzyme-inducing AEDs such as phenobarbitone, phenytoin and carbamazepine, it will be difficult to predict the strength of this effect in an individual patient. Furthermore, there can be rather unexpected drug-drug interactions. Finally pharmacodynamic (or pharmacokinetic?) tolerance to the effect of an AED could be unnoticed.

As a measure of drug action the concentration in blood can be measured (AED-level). For most drugs there exists a "therapeutic range." In clinical practice AED-levels are generally used to determine drug choice and replacement. J.W.A. Meijer (1991) has investigated the strategy of sixteen prescribing doctors in the Instituut voor Epilepsiebestrijding, Heemstede: they were confronted with blood levels below or above the so-called therapeutic ranges (see Table 1 for results). Primarily it shows differences in use of this laboratory information between the clinicians. Levels above therapeutic range proved to be more alarming than levels below. The majority consider

Table 1. Strategy of 16 prescribing doctors (IVE, Heemstede) confronted with aed-levels below or above "therapeutic ranges"

	Strategy					
	+		±		−	
	Below	Above	Below	Above	Below	Above
Repeat assay	1	5	14	10	1	1
Always increase/decrease dosage	–	–	1	6	15	10
Increase if not seizure free; decrease if toxic signs	15	12	1	4	–	–
Wait for clinical signs	13	5	3	11	–	–
Change formulation or regimen	–	–	10	16	6	–
Check prescription or compliance	8	6	7	7	1	3
Do additional pharmacological investigations	–	–	12	12	4	4

Number of doctors who took action specified in column I, if anti-epileptic druglevel is above or below the "therapeutic range" (Meijer 1991).
+ = always action; ± = generally/sometimes action; − = never action

the AED blood levels as a means to sanction their opinion: if a patient shows side-effects a high blood level confirms this. Some clinicians advocate that they do not treat blood levels but patients.

Drug Withdrawal

Since the 1980's, when patients are seizure-free for two or three years, it is general practice to try to withdraw AED treatment. Overweg (1985) found that only a combination of clinical variables (age at last seizure, blood levels and number of drugs) proved to be predictive of outcome. The risk of relapse diminished with increasing number of drugs, regardless of the other two variables. A given blood level is associated with greater efficacy if it is achieved with one drug then if two or three are used. However, it is unclear whether these results can be generalized because this study was performed in a tertiary referral hospital.

RESEARCH

Standardized measurement of efficacy and toxicity of therapy is necessary, especially in research. Unlike in daily clinical practice, where the patient with epileptic seizures seeks help, in research it is the doctor who is in need of epileptic patients to participate in a clinical trial. The doctor will select patients with a specific type of seizures and/or a certain seizure frequency, or based on their age (no children or seniors), sex and level of intelligence. Patients with a history of allergic reactions are usually not eligible to enter a pharmaceutical trial. Generally very little is known about pharmacokinetic and dynamic interactions of the new drug with existing AEDs nor about possible side-effects in patients with epilepsy. Colleagues can not help with information on the drug and experience with the new drug is obviously lacking. Thus, the situation in clinical trials is quite different compared to general practice, although the parameters for evaluation of efficacy and toxicity of the new AED is the same as for the already registered drugs. The unpredictability of seizures, together with general precipitating factors such as stress, night-sleep deprivation, and fever, make it difficult to evaluate efficacy of an experimental drug in the relatively short time course of the trial.

Time is limited in research projects for several reasons: the burden for patients as well as doctors (extra visits, additional examinations) and budgets will set a limit. Even more in clinical research than in clinical practice, standardization of methods is necessary in order to be able to compare results within and between patients. Clinimetrics may be of great help.

Acknowledgement. This work was supported by a grant of CLEO-NEF (Netherlands).

REFERENCES

M.J. Eadie and J.H. Tyrer. Anticonvulsant Therapy. Ed.: Churchill Livingstone, third edition, 1989, page 16.

J.W.A. Meijer. Knowledge, attitude and practice in antiepileptic drug monitoring. Acta Neurol. Scand. (1991) suppl. no. 134, vol. 83:75–76.

J. Overweg. Withdrawal of antiepileptic drugs in seizure-free adult patients: prediction of outcome. Thesis, Rodopi, Amsterdam (1985): page 160.

E.H. Reynolds and S.D. Shorvon. Single drug or multiple drug therapy for epilepsy? The Lancet, February 28, 1981:507.

INDIVIDUALIZATION OF ANTIEPILEPTIC DRUG THERAPY

Y.A. Hekster, Ph.D.,[1] D.J.P. Wijsman, M.D.,[2] E.W. Wuis, Ph.D.,[1]
T.B. Vree, Ph.D.,[1] and H. Meinardi, M.D., Ph.D.[2]

[1]Department of Clinical Pharmacy
[2]Institute for Neurology
University Hospital Nijmegen
P.O. Box 9101
6500 HB Nijmegen
The Netherlands

INTRODUCTION

The ultimate goal of anti-epileptic drug (AED) therapy is to enable the patient to live a normal life. The usual approach is to maximize seizure control and to minimize the risk of adverse effects [Pugh and Garnett 1991]. After careful consideration of the nature of the epilepsy, chronic AED treatment should be started. The initial choice of a particular drug depends upon the type of disorder and on individual patient characteristics. Since large variations in AED pharmacokinetics have been observed, it is not possible to start the drug of choice with individualized, patient-tailored regimen. Individualization takes patient characteristics and drug characteristics into consideration, and tries to integrate these issues to obtain the most rational dosage schedule for that patient. Before such a step can be made, and individualization is obtained, drug regimen should be based on data obtained from groups of patients that have been treated for the particular seizure disorder with that particular drug. For that reason, the initial dose regimen for any patient is based on population pharmacokinetic data. Population pharmacokinetics can be defined as the study of the variability in plasma drug concentrations between individuals when standard dosage regimens are administered [Aarons 1991]. These studies assess the influence of patient's variabilities, such as age, gender, race, pregnancy, liver and kidney function, on drug kinetics. In addition, drug characteristics such as metabolism, stereoselectivity and activity, drug-drug and drug-food interactions and, the influence of co-medication [Eadie 1991] are considered. Another factor influencing pharmacokinetic properties of a drug, includes the disease state itself [Encinas et al 1992, Vree et al 1989, Yukawa et al 1992]. For instance it has been observed that serum albumin binding of phenytoin during

Quantitative Assessment in Epilepsy Care, Edited by H. Meinardi et al.
Plenum Press, New York, 1993

109

Table 1. Evaluation of the treatment process

Patient	Choice of Treatment	Outcome Assessment
A) Individual Factors	• Treatment objective	• Seizure activity
• Age, gender	• Disease severity	• Seizure severity
• Pregnancy	• Drug(s) + doses	• Adverse reactions
• Organ functions	• Duration	• Quality of life
• Race	• Referral period	• Quality of care
• Size (length, kg)	• Mono vs. poly therapy	
• Life style		
• Compliance		
B) Disease Factors		
• Co-medication		
• Organ function		

monotherapy and polytherapy with other AEDs differs, varying from no effect on binding (phenobarbitone), a small decrease in effect (carbamazepine) or a statistically significant decrease (valproic acid) [Pospisil and Perlik 1992]. Changes in binding directly influence the fraction of unbound or free (active) drug, making individualization in dose necessary. In addition, changes in a patient's health state, his compliance to drug therapy, the start of new drugs with unknown drug interactions etc. make individualization on a continuous basis even more important. Individualization can potentially improve the quality of patient care by improving safety and efficacy of drug therapy and is essential for drugs with an erratic or unpredictable dose-response curve. A number of drugs used in epilepsy care fulfil these requirements.

In epilepsy, the effect of a drug on seizure activity can be demonstrated using an outcome parameter. Nowadays, in this clinimetric approach, the severity of the seizure is also taken into account in addition to many other factors such as side effects, and plasma concentrations [Baker et al 1991, Cramer et al 1983, Duncan and Sanders 1991, Wijsman et al 1991]. The choice of a particular treatment approach is a continuous process and is based upon patient criteria, the process of decision of the choice of treatment and output assessment using measuring parameters shown in table 1.

This manuscript describes drugs and patient factors that may influence the measured plasma concentration. The discussion focuses on clinimetric modulation factors made when plasma concentrations are not within the therapeutic range.

CLINIMETRICS AND PLASMA CONCENTRATIONS

In the design of clinimetrics for epilepsy, rating scales have been developed both for research activities and for the clinical setting [Cramer et al 1983, Wijsman et al 1991]. In clinimetric evaluations, a final composite score is determined which gives an indication of the patient's "health" state. Several factors have an impact on the seizure rating such as the presence of an aura, clustering of seizures, lack of sleep and alcohol intake. These factors are used to modulate rating scores as is the level of the plasma concentration.

Cramer et al (1983) reduce the score by 70 percent when the drug serum concentration is subtherapeutic or by 20 percent when low therapeutic serum drug levels are measured. When a toxic level is encountered (especially with side effects), the dose is reduced and reevaluation takes place at a time when the concentration is within the therapeutic range.

Wijsman et al (1991) use similar modulating factors; they have included a modulation factor for phenytoin drug levels which are above the therapeutic range. Modulations affect the final composite score, indicating whether a patient is scored as clinically good, acceptable, or unacceptable.

FACTORS INFLUENCING THE MEASURED CONCENTRATION

As discussed above, corrections are made for a plasma concentration which is not in the therapeutic range. However, it should be asked what plasma concentration itself means. It is generally agreed that plasma concentration reflects the concentration in the biophase at the receptor, but which receptor is responsible for the specific types of epilepsy (ies)? Also receptor populations change (as a self defence) due to the presence of AED, occupying receptor areas while body function must be maintained. In addition, several factors can influence the measured concentration and these factors can be separated into drug- and in patient characteristics. A formal discussion should take place about their relevance in assessing the modulation percentage of the seizure score.

DRUG CHARACTERISTICS

Sample Time

Therapeutic Drug Monitoring (TDM) will result in the measurement of a particular value of a drug. Whether this value is appropriate and reliable, depends upon several factors. Much attention has been focused in the past on the reliability of the technique used for the monitoring. This will not be discussed here nor will discussions take place about the quality of the sampling time. (Pugh and Garnett 1991). It has become clear that in many cases drug levels have been monitored before the steady state concentration for the drug had been reached. Also the sampling timing in relation to drug dosing is an interfering factor. Up to 74 percent of samples for phenytoin were inappropriately taken [Levine et al 1988]. Modulations based upon inappropriate sampling times are not rational.

Drug Stereoisomers

Many antiepileptic drugs are administered as racemic mixtures (Table 2). Measuring of total drug levels (sum of the individual enantiomer levels) may therefore produce non-

Table 2. Antiepileptic drugs

Drug Administered as Racemic Mixture	Achiral Drug	Achiral Drug with Active Chiral Metabolite
• Ethosuximide	• Carbamazepine	• Oxcarbazepine
• Mephenytoin	• Phenytoin	
• Mesuximide	• Valproate	
• Methylphenobarbital		
• Phenobarbital		
• Primidon		
• Thiopental		
• Vigabatrin		

sensical pharmacokinetic parameters. Enantiomers may have different pharmacological properties and differ in their kinetics, thus individual drug enantiomer levels must be determined. The technology needed to separate and quantitate drug enantiomers is advancing rapidly. For methylphenobarbital, mephenytoin, phenobarbital, and pentobarbital (a metabolite of thiopental) stereoselective pharmacokinetics have been demonstrated, but the clinical implications are yet unclear [Hall et al 1987, Krstulovic 1989, Lim and Hooper 1989], because of the unavailability of the chiral products for clinical use. Studies should be carried out with pure isomers of the drug to assess their intrinsic activity and to learn how the patient responds to this activity, but these are rarely performed.

Extra clinical benefit is not obtained by monitoring individual enantiomer levels of vigabatrin or the oxcarbazepine metabolite. For vigabatrin plasma drug levels are not related to the clinical effect and population kinetics do not make sense [Schechter 1987]; for oxcarbazepine, both enantiomeric forms of the metabolite have anticonvulsant properties [Schütz et al 1986]. Thus in TDM, one should always be aware of the problems that may arise from the existence of enantiomeric forms or enantiomeric (active) metabolites, and their intrinsic activities. Modulation of treatment scores based on enantiomer drug levels, should be investigated.

Protein Binding

AED's are highly bound to albumin and several factors can alter this binding. Since only the free fraction is considered as pharmacologically active, it seems reasonable to measure only this fraction. When there is no covalent binding, protein binding may be considered as storage and transport function of the drug. However, measurement of the unbound concentration is not without problems. Because of the high percentage plasma protein binding, only a low free concentration will be found, and it is questionable whether "simple" assay techniques will become available for rapid routine measurement. Due to the lack of clinical experience, a clear cut therapeutic range for the free fractions is at present unavailable and in practice it is seldom assessed. Furthermore, the relationship between the total concentration, the free fraction and the clinical effect is far from clear. It is known that concomitant prescribed drugs can alter the binding of drugs highly bound to albumin and other proteins. This means that the degree of protein binding can change during treatment. Obviously these issues require further investigation.

Drug Metabolism

In general therapeutic drug monitoring measures the active parent compound. However, all of the commonly used anticonvulsants are extensively metabolised before excretion takes place. It is well known that some of the metabolites are pharmacologically active. This activity can be expressed in terms of drug efficacy and of drug toxicity (adverse drug reactions), as has been shown, for example, for metabolites of valproic acid, carbamazepine, phenytoin, etc..

Recently, the issue of the formation of active metabolites of anticonvulsant drugs in relation to their pharmacokinetic and therapeutic significance has been reviewed [Eadie 1991]. Monitoring of parent drug alone is not the goal in TDM, and is not sufficient. This should be regarded as a pre-TDM approach. Metabolites must be included in the overall discussion about the dose-effects–quality of life relationship. How the formation of active metabolites and their concentrations should be included into the modulation factors, is open for further discussion.

Drug Elimination

If a patient does not respond to a 'normal' dose based upon population pharmacokinetics, a plasma drug level is measured and the dose accordingly adjusted. This adjustment should be carefully approached, as has been discussed under sample time. Uniform doses of drugs in different patients can lead to large variation in concentrations measured and in the intensity of effect. Much of this individual variation can be explained by variation in drug metabolism and drug elimination. Therapeutic drug monitoring is based upon this concept: the patient's dose is individualized to achieve a desired concentration of the parent drug in the plasma (the 'therapeutic' level of the individual patient). It has already been discussed that active metabolites can interfere with the finding of the therapeutic range. Individualization based upon patient's own data is the current practice in drug therapy for epilepsy. A number of techniques have been described to estimate individual drug doses in clinical practice. These techniques vary from simple graphic methods based on one [Martin et al 1977], two or more steady state plasma levels at different daily doses [Armijo and Cavada 1991, Pryka et al 1991], to personal computers.

PATIENT CHARACTERISTICS

From a pharmacokinetic point of view a large number of patient characteristics can interfere with the fate of drugs in the body. It is well known that the functioning of organs plays a crucial role in drug metabolism (liver + isoenzyme composition) and drug elimination (kidney), and thus has a major effect on the concentration that is measured in TDM. Compliance factors also contribute substantially to unexpected drug levels. Patient

.compliance is a major problem for the assessment of success in treatment strategy in epileptic patients. It should be kept in mind, however, that when composite scores in patients with severely reduced kidney or liver function are modulated and compared with results which are obtained in "normal" epileptic patients, or in non-compliant patients, biased results can be obtained. It might be better to group specific patients together and introduce group modulation factors which could serve as a more appropriate basis for modulating the composite score. This concept should be discussed in future clinimetric research protocols. Differences were found in a preliminary analysis of patients treated with either mono- or polytherapy, to examine differences between those groups. How blood levels for polytherapy can be included into the score technique is still unclear.

Mono- versus Polytherapy

The question whether a relationship exists between clinical severity and choice for polypharmacy, has recently been under investigation. The following data were obtained from 105 patients studied at the Instituut voor Epilepsiebestrijding (Utrecht). Dependent on the treatment objective (seizure remission, individual treatment or other goals) some preliminary results in the relationship of mono- and poly pharmacy and obtained effects are given in Table 3. The average clinical severity, as scored by the treating physician on a 7-point scale (0 good, 7 severe), and is shown in brackets. The objective seizure remission is mostly assigned to new patients, in whom efficacy is most important. In "individual treatment" chronic patients are given, in whom further seizure remission could not be achieved. A balance is looked for between efficacy and toxicity. The group of "other treatment goals" consists of patients that show absolute intractability, etc. In these patients efforts are made to minimize side effects, while maximum therapy is prescribed.

Table 3. Number of patients in relation to drugs and effect

Treatment Objective		Mono-pharmacy*	Poly-pharmacy*	Total*
I.	Seizure remission			
	Effective: Yes	18 (2)	14 (2)	32 (2)
	No	0	3 (2)	3 (2)
	Total	18	17	35
II.	Individual treatment risk-benefit balance			
	Effective: Yes	6 (3)	22 (3)	28 (3)
	No	4 (4)	16 (3)	20 (3)
	Total	10	38	48
III.	Other goals			
	Effective: Yes	1 (4)	2 (4)	3 (4)
	No	2 (6)	17 (5)	19 (5)
	Total	3	19	22

*Number (severity score)

In 63 out of 105, effective treatment conforming to the subjective objectives of the physician was obtained. It can be concluded that when remission is the objective, a majority of patients can be treated successfully with monotherapy. Where individualization is the treatment objective, a majority of patients are treated with polytherapy, possibly caused by the different types of epilepsy. In those patients in whom optimal efficacy of drug treatment has not yet been realized, a worse clinical severity rating is noted. This is suggestive of a relationship between the severity of the epilepsy and the choice of poly therapy.

CONCLUSION

Clinimetrics is a new discipline that enables assessing the assessment of the most rational treatment for a particular patient. Data may be obtained from groups of patients which can help in making individually based choices. Scores provide a means to assess whether treatment is successful and can be used as parameters in comparative studies. When modulation is applied to plasma concentrations outside the therapeutic range, it should be borne in mind that a large number of variables can interfere with the outcome. These variables should be studied in more detail before clear-cut decisions are made. In the field of clinimetrics this is highly relevant, since drugs play such a major role in the treatment of patients with epilepsy.

Acknowledgement. This work was supported by a grant of CLEO-NEF (Netherlands).

REFERENCES

Aarons L. Population pharmacokinetics: theory and practice. British Journal of Clinical Pharmacology 1991; 32: 669– 70

Armijo J.A. and Cavada E. Graphic estimation of phenytoin dose in adults and children. Therapeutic Drug Monitoring 1991; 13: 507–10

Baker G.A., Smith D.F., Dewey M, Morrow J, Crawford P.M., Chadwick D.W. The development of a seizure severity scale as an outcome measure in epilepsy. Epilepsy Research 1991; 8: 245–51

Cramer J.A. Smith D.B., Mattson, R.H. et al. A method of quantification for the evaluation of antiepileptic drug therapy. Neurology 1983; 33 (suppl 1): 26–37

Duncan J.S. and Sanders J.W.A.S. The Chalfont Seizure Severity scale. Journal of Neurology, Neurosurgery and Psychiatry 1991; 54: 873–6

Eadie M.J. Formation of active metabolites of anticonvulsant drugs. Clinical Pharmacokinetics 1991; 21: 27–41

Encinas M.P., Santos Buelga D, Alonso González A.C., Garcioa Sáanches M.J. and Dominguez-Gil Hurlé A. Influence of length of treatment on the interaction between phenobarbital and phenytoin. Journal of Clinical Pharmacy and Therapeutics 1992; 17: 49–50

Hall S.D., Guengerich F.P., Branch R.A., Wilkinson G.R., Characterization and inhibition of mephenytoin 4-hydroxylase activity in human liver microsomes. Journal of Pharmacology and Experimental Therapy 1987; 240: 216–22

Krstulovic A.M. (ed.) Chiral separations by HPLC, Ellis Horwood, New York, 1989.

Levine M, McCollom R, Chang T et al. Evaluation of serum phenytoin monitoring in an acute care setting. Therapeutic Drug Monitoring 1988; 10: 50–7

Lim W.H., Hooper W.D. Stereoselective metabolism and pharmacokinetics of racemic methylphenobarbital in humans. Drug Metabolism Disposition 1989; 17: 212–7

Martin E, Tozer T.N., Sheiner L.B., Riegelman S. The clinical pharmacokinetics of phenytoin. Journal of Pharmacokinetics and Biopharmaceutics 1977; 5: 579–96

Pospisil J and Perlik E. Binding parameters of phenytoin during monotherapy and polytherapy. International Journal of Clinical Pharmacology Therapy and Toxicology 1992; 30: 24–28

Pryka R.D., Rodvold K.A. and Erdman S.M. An updated comparison of drug dosing methods, Part I. Clinical Pharmacokinetics 1991; 20: 209–217

Pugh C.B. and Garnett W.R. Current issues in the treatment of epilepsy. Clinical Pharmacy 1991; 10: 335–58

Schechter P.J. Clinical pharmacology of vigabatrin. British Journal of Clinical Pharmacology 1989; 27 Suppl 1:19S–22S

Schütz H, Feldman K.F., Faigle J.W., Kriemler H-P, Winkler T. The metabolism of ^{14}C-oxcarbazepine in man. Xenobiotica 1986; 16: 769–78

Vree T.B., Shimoda M., Driessen J.J., Guelen P.J.M., Janssen T.J.,Termond E.F.S., Van Dalen R., Hafkenscheid J.C.M., and Dirksen M.S.C. Decreased plasma albumin concentration results in increased volume of distribution and decreased elimination of midazolam in intensive care patients. Clinical Pharmacology and Therapeutics 1989; 46: 537–44

Wijsman D.J.P., Hekster Y.A., Keijser A., Renier W.O. and Meinardi H. Clinimetrics and Epilepsy Care. Pharmaceutisch Weekblad [Scientific Edition] 1991; 13: 182–188

Yukawa E, Suzuki A, Higuchi S and Aoyama T. Influence of age and co-medication on steady-state carbamazepine serum level-dose ratios in Japanese paediatric patients. Journal of Clinical Pharmacy and Therapeutics 1992; 17: 65–9

ON THE REPORTING OF ADVERSE DRUG EVENTS

M.W. Lammers, M.D. and H. Meinardi, M.D., Ph.D.

Institute of Neurology
University Hospital St. Radboud
Catholic University Nijmegen
Nijmegen, The Netherlands

INTRODUCTION

In this paper only dose dependent adverse drug events will be discussed.

Adverse drug events are by definition a problem in efficacy studies. In studies of anti-epileptic drugs an additional problem arises. As the desired effect of an anti-epileptic drug is the suppression of a paroxysmal and unpredictable event, titration to reach an optimal dose is not readily practicable using the desired effect parameter.

It is commonly accepted to substitute the occurrence of adverse effects as end-point minus one for the titration phase. Of course this poses a problem with respect to the reporting of the occurrence of side effects. Proper policy would be to disregard side-effects elicited during a titration phase. The possibility to monitor serumlevels did offer a way out of this problem by choosing a serumlevel below the "toxic range" as first end-point of titration. However, recent anti-epileptic drugs show little or no correlation between serumlevels and pharmacodynamic properties of these drugs. Examples are vigabatrin and milacemide. If adverse effects are only to be reported during steady state and in relation to seizure suppression the whimsical nature of adverse events may become a confounding factor. As was shown by the epileptologists from Milan[1] adverse effects may or may not disappear spontaneously. There are no systematic studies about the pathophysiology of this tolerance phenomenon. However, there are anecdotal reports of people withdrawn from anti-epileptic drug treatment who felt much improved even though they did not have any formal complaints about adverse effects prior to withdrawal.

In drug-trial reports the methods section often contains little information about the procedures with respect to the evaluation of adverse drug events. For example in a recent paper by Reynolds et al.[2] on a study of vigabatrin it is stated that "Efficacy was assessed

Quantitative Assessment in Epilepsy Care, Edited by H. Meinardi et al.
Plenum Press, New York, 1993

117

Table 1. Adverse events leading to study withdrawl

Patient	Days with GVG	Adverse Event
1	14	Headache, abdominal pain
2	23	Depression
3	56	Increased lability of mood, unsteady gait, disturbed sleep
4	56	Headache, nocturia
5	56	Dizziness
6	56	Depression, swollen breasts
7	56	Depression, confusion

GVG, vigabatrin
Reproduced with permission from Reynolds, E.H. et al. Open, double-blind and long-term study of vigabatrin in chronic epilepsy. *Epilepsia* 32:530, 1991

by seizure frequency, calculated from patient's diaries. Possible adverse events were recorded from patient's spontaneous reports, responses to questions, physical examination and haematologic/metabolic investigations (blood count, urea electrolytes, sugar, calcium liver function) performed on each clinic visit." Subsequently the account of the statistical analysis in this paper only refers to the analysis of changes in seizure frequency. From the discussions on withdrawal and on adverse events in this paper it is clear that some criterion was used called "unacceptable adverse event." However, no description of that criterion was presented in the paper. The specific adverse events leading to withdrawal were tabulated as follows. (table 1) However, headache and depression were also seen in other patients without subsequent withdrawal from the trial as witnessed from the summary of adverse events presented in that paper. (table 2)

In order to obtain an assessment of the present reporting of adverse events it was decided to make a limited but systematic overview.

METHODS

The screening of the literature was restricted to the official journal of the International League Against Epilepsy Epilepsia for the years 1987 through 1991. All papers reporting on aspects of the treatment of epilepsy with anti-epileptic drugs were included. In total 118 papers were screened. Twenty-two papers presented quantitative data. These papers will be further analyzed in the result section.

RESULTS

Twenty papers were specifically concerned with adverse effects. Five papers dealt with the effects of anti-epileptic drugs on cognition.[3,4,5,6,7] The paper by Reinvang et al.[5] also measured subjective symptoms of discomfort i.e. fatigue, headache, nausea, incoordination, diplopia and blurred vision using a visual analogue scale. However, the reported level of discomfort was generally very low. Four papers also used the quantitative data of serumlevels [3,4,5,7] One paper by Robertson et al.[8] used depression rating scales in the assessment of depression in epilepsy. Twelve papers were concerned with other specific adverse effects, which usually are reported in a global manner like the problem of rashes,[9] edema,[10] or are intrinsically quantitative, because they concern laboratory measurements like levels of lipids, vitamins and proteins.[11] These authors also discussed morphology of liver biopsy specimens which were, however, not judged in a quantitative manner. M. Berg et al. looked at changes in the folate levels after taking phenytoin.[12] Jouko I.T. Isojärvi et al. looked in two studies at sexhormone levels in male and female patients[13,14] Gough et al. studied bilirubin levels[15] and two paper were concerned with the changes in immunoglobulin levels[16,17] Goyle et al. looked at mutagenicity of anti-epileptic drugs measuring the mitotic index and sister chromatid exchange[18] and W. Fletjer studied the cytogenic effects of AED using the same parameters.[19] L. Carenini et al. studied SSEP (somatosensory evoked potentials) changes.[20] One paper was a comprehensive study of side effects, both adverse and favourable comparing five major anti-epileptic drugs.[21]

Two papers concerned efficacy studies of anti-epileptic drugs. Koeppen et al. compared clobazam with placebo and used mood scales and a global assessment of adverse events as "not significantly interfering with patient's functioning," "significantly interfering" and "outweighing therapeutic effect".[22] Woo et al.[23] studied the change of recurrence of seizures in groups of patients in remission though on a dosage of anti-epileptic drugs producing serumlevels in the sub-therapeutic range. Part of the patients

Table 2. Summary of adverse events

| Adverse Event | Baseline Phase (n = 33) | Open Phase (n = 33) | Double Blind Phase | | Long-term Phase | |
			Active (n =10)	Placebo (n = 10)	6–12 mo (n = 17)	12–18 (n = 17)
Drowsiness	9	17	2	0	2	0
Depression/irritibility	2	8	0	0	0	2
Headache	1	6	0	1	0	1
Behavior disturbance	0	3	0	1	0	1
Confusion	0	3	0	0	1	0
Increased micturition	0	3	0	0	0	0
Dizziness	0	2	1	0	1	1
Increased appetite and weight	0	2	0	0	3	2

Reproduced with permission from Reynolds, E.H. et al. Open, double-blind and long-term study of vigabatrin in chronic epilepsy. *Epilepsia* 32:530, 1991 received additional doses in order to increase the serum level to the therapeutic range, while the other part was maintained on a subtherapeutic level as before. They assessed their patients using systemic toxicity and neurologic toxicity scales modified from Cramer et al.[24]

The other papers screened used no quantitative measures in assessing adverse effects. In most drug efficacy studies authors described the number or percentage of patients, who suffered from adverse effects of the medication. In some papers case reports were used when describing rare adverse events.

DISCUSSION

Studies about the adverse effects of antiepileptic drugs rarely use quantitative data in order to describe the adverse effects. In studies of the efficacy or toxicity of antiepileptic drugs the adverse events are rarely described according to severity but in most cases according to frequency or number of patients with adverse effects of medication. When quantitative data has been used to describe adverse effects, the adverse effects studied were intrinsically quantified, because they were based upon laboratory findings. Also when assessing cognitive functions standardised tests are available. Semi-quantification is variably used, but then the categories are generally poorly characterised, like *mild, moderate* or *severe* with no explanation of what exactly is meant by these terms.

When quantification scales for adverse effects are applied, most authors develop new rating scales and rarely are rating scales of other authors used. For this reason comparing results of different studies concerned with adverse events is difficult. Especially as the complaints suggesting adverse drug effects sometimes are already present before the drug under evaluation has been administered, a more quantitative comparison of the two phases would be in place. The lack of detail in the reports on adverse effects is also reflected in the reviews of the subject (Meinardi and Stoel, Meinardi, Schmidt.)[25,26,27]

While dose dependent toxicity may prevent full use of the seizure suppressing capacity of the compound, idiosyncratic adverse effects can necessitate complete abandon of the drug. Here again in the past little or no use has been made of quantitative presentation of the associated problem. Yet it is well recognised that the severity of idiosyncratic reactions is not always the same. At least from the literature, it is not clear whether for example granulocytopenia should be considered a mild form of agranulocytosis or whether allergic exanthemas are abortive cases of exfoliative dermatitis.

Consensus on quantification of adverse events for clinical symptoms as well as for laboratory findings and other standardised tests, will be useful in order to be able to compare studies on this topic.

CONCLUSIONS

Apart from symptoms characterised by changes in clinical chemistry or haematological data, very little quantification is used to report about the adverse effects of antiepileptic drugs as witnessed by a review of papers which appeared over the past five years in the official journal of the International League Against Epilepsy "Epilepsia."

Acknowledgement. This work was supported by a grant of CLEO-NEF (Netherlands).

REFERENCES

1. Collaborative Group for Epidemiology of Epilepsy, 1988, Adverse reactions to antiepileptic drugs: a follow-up study of 355 patients with chronic antiepileptic drug treatment. *Epilepsia* 29:787.
2. Reynolds, E.H., Ring, H.A., Farr, I.N., Heller, A.J. and Elwes, R.D.C., 1991, Open, double-blind and long-term study of vigabatrin in chronic epilepsy. *Epilepsia* 32:530.
3. Berent S., Sackellares J.C., Giordani B., Wagner, J.G., Donofrio, P.D. and Abou-Khalil, B., 1987, Zonisamide (CT-912) and cognition: results from preliminary study. *Epilepsia* 28:61.
4. Aman, M.G., Werry, J.S., Paxton, J.W. and Turbott, S.H. 1987, Effect of sodium valproate on psychomotor performance in children as a function of dose fluctuations in concentration and diagnosis. *Epilepsia* 28:115
5. Reinvang, I., Bjartveit, S., Johannessen, S.I., Hagen, O.P., Larsch, S., Fagerthun, H. and Gjerstad, L., 1991, Cognitive function and time-of-day variation in serum carbamazepine concentration in epileptic patients treated with monotherapy. *Epilepsia* 32:116.
6. Mitchell, W.G. and Chavez, J.M. 1987, Carbamazepine versus phenobarbital for partial onset seizures in children. *Epilepsia* 28:56.
7. Aldenkamp, A.P., Alpherts, W.C.J., Moerland, M.C., Ottevanger, N. and Van Parijs, J.A.P., 1987, Controlled release carbamazepine: cognitive side effects in patients with epilepsy. *Epilepsia* 28:507.
8. Robertson, M.M., Trimble, M.R. and Townsend, H.R.A., 1987, Phenomenology of depression in epilepsy. *Epilepsia* 28:364.
9. Pelekanos, J., Camfield, P., Camfield, C., and Gordon, K., 1991, Allergic rash due to antiepileptic drugs; clinical features and management. *Epilepsia* 32:554.
10. Ettinger, A., Moshe, S. and Shinnar, S., 1990, Edema associated with long-term valproate therapy. *Epilepsia* 31:211.
11. Dastur, D.K., and Dave, U.P., 1987, Effect of prolonged anticonvulsant medication in epileptic patients: serum lipids, vitamins B6, B12, and folic acid, proteins, and fine structure of liver. Epilepsia 28:147.
12. Berg, M.J., Fincham, R.W., Ebert, B.E. and Schottelius, D., 1988, Decrease of serum folates in healthy male volunteers taking phenytoin. *Epilepsia* 29:67.
13. Isojärvi, J.I.T., Pakarinen, A.J. and Myllylä, V.V., 1989, Effects of carbamazepine on the hypothalamic-pituitary-gonadal axis in male patients with epilepsy: a prospective study. Epilepsia 30:446.
14. Isojärvi, J.I.T., 1990, Serum steroid hormones and pituitary function in female epileptic patients during carbamazepine therapy. *Epilepsia* 31:438
15. Gough, H., Goggin, T., Crowley M. and Callaghan, N., 1989, Serum bilirubin levels with antiepileptic drugs. *Epilepsia* 30:597.
16. Gilhus, N.E. and Tor, L., 1988, Carbamazepine: effect on IgG subclasses in epileptic patients. *Epilepsia* 29:317.
17. Pacifici, R., Paris, L., Di Carlo, S., 1991, Immunologic aspects of carbamazepine treatment in epileptic patients. *Epilepsia* 32:122.
18. Goyle, S., Maurya, A.K., Kailash, S. and Maheshwari, M.C., 1987, Mutagenic risk in epileptic patients before and after anticonvulsant therapy. *Epilepsia* 28:81.
19. Fletjer W.J., Astemborski, J.A., Hassel, T.M. and Cohen, M.M., 1989, Cytogenic effects of phenytoin and/or carbamazepine on human peripheral leukocytes. *Epilepsia* 30:374.
20. Carenini L., Bottachi, E., Camerlingo, M., D'Allesandro, G. and Mamoli, A., 1988, Carbamazepine does not affect short latency somatosensory evoked potentials: a longitudinal study in newly diagnosed epilepsy. *Epilepsia* 29:145
21. Herranz, J.L., Arinijo, J.A. and Arteaga R., 1988, Clinical side effects of phenobarbital, primidone, phenytoin, carbamazepine and valproate during monotherapy in children. *Epilepsia* 29:794.

22. Koeppen, D., Baruzzi, A., Capozza, M., et al., 1987, Clobazam in therapy-resistant patients with partial epilepsy: a double-blind placebo-controlled crossover study. *Epilepsia* 28:495.

23. Woo, E, Chan, Y.M., Yu, Y.L., Chan, Y.W. and Huang, C.Y., 1988, If a well-stabilized epileptic patient has a sub-therapeutic antiepileptic drug level, should the dose be increased? *Epilepsia* 29:129.

24. Cramer, J.A., Smith, D.B., Mattson, R.H., et al., 1983, A method of quantification for the evaluation of antiepileptic drug therapy. Neurology 33 (supl 1): 26.

25. Meinardi H, Stoel L.M.K., 1974, Side-effects of antiepileptic drugs, Handbook of Neurology vol 15, p.705–738, ed. Magnus O, Lorentz de Haas A.M., North Holland Publ. Cie.

26. Meinardi H., Side effects of new drugs and new side effects of old drugs. 1980, In: Canger R., Angeleri F., and Penry J.K., eds.: Advances in epileptology. p.391–398, Raven Press New York.

27. Schmidt D., Adverse effects of anti-epileptic drugs, 1982 Raven Press.

QUANTITATIVE ASSESSMENT OF ADVERSE DRUG EFFECTS

Richard H. Mattson, M.D. and Joyce A. Cramer, B.S.

Department of Veterans Affairs Medical Center
950 Campbell Avenue
West Haven, Connecticut 06516, U.S.A.

INTRODUCTION

Antiepileptic drugs possess the properties of decreasing frequency and severity of seizures to variable degrees. For many seizure and epilepsy types, seizure control is effective at modest drug dose (Mattson, 1989, Heller et al., 1989, Bourgeois et al., 1987). However, those patients whose seizure control cannot be realized by any single or combination of drugs often need to have their dose increased to a point of maximal tolerance as evidenced by undesirable adverse effects. In fact, while the choice among major antiepileptic drugs is theoretically based on efficacy, the results of the VA Epilepsy Cooperative Study and other trials have demonstrated that most drugs are similarly efficacious, so that selection of a specific drug for an individual can be based largely on expected side effects (Mattson et al., 1984, 1985, 1989, 1992).

Definition of an Adverse Effect

An adverse effect is a deleterious or unintended outcome caused by use of therapeutic doses of an agent such as an antiepileptic drug. No drug is without side effects, albeit some subtle factor. The risk:benefit ratio of using a therapeutic drug is based on the assumption that the efficacy of the agent in controlling the disorder, (i.e., epilepsy), outweighs the risk or severity of potential adverse effects caused by the use of the agent.

At the present time, in most studies of antiepileptic drugs, characterizations of adverse effects are descriptive or nominal in type. For example, barbiturates are often said to be associated with sedation, carbamazepine with visual disturbances, phenytoin with incoordination, and valproate with weight gain. These terms do not convey information about

Quantitative Assessment in Epilepsy Care, Edited by H. Meinardi et al.
Plenum Press, New York, 1993

123

frequency or severity which might allow definition and interpretation of the importance of the problem. The absence of well-defined methods to identify, record and quantify adverse effects makes it difficult to clearly characterize them, particularly relative to seizure control. Such quantification is particularly important in clinical trials.

CLINIMETRIC ASSESSMENTS

Limitations in assessing clinical outcomes have been well-recognized for most medical problems and many attempts have been made to standardize and quantitate clinical measures. The term "clinimetrics" (Feinstein, 1987) is defined as a system of quantification of clinical status, medical syndromes, or clinical events. Feinstein has reviewed these principles and illustrated how a scientific approach can allow clinical "impressions" to be defined in numerical measures (see chapter by Feinstein).

Recognizing the need for detailed measurement methodology during the design of a multicentre study of antiepileptic drugs in the mid 1970's, the VA Cooperative Study Group undertook the development of a study designed to measure frequency and severity of seizures, and adverse effects, and an overall composite (global) outcome. After development, this system was utilized in a six-year study (1978–1985) of efficacy and toxicity involving 622 patients with epilepsy treated with carbamazepine, phenobarbital, phenytoin, or primidone. The second multicentre study (1985–1991) of 480 patients compared carbamazepine and valproate in a similar study design. The original rating scales were modified to define adverse effects expected with use of these two drugs.

RATING SCALE DEVELOPMENT: GENERAL CHARACTERISTICS

Development of adverse effect rating scales requires identification of anticipated effects. The most elementary type of rating is a simple listing of type of an adverse event and frequency of occurrence. Increasing levels of specificity are often possible and desirable, with further grouping into a classification as systemic or neurotoxic. Laboratory test changes are a separate category or subdivisions of the primary systemic categories (e.g., liver function tests, electrolytes). A major subgroup of adverse neurotoxic effects are outcomes of detailed neuropsychological assessments of cognition, affect, and mood. Adverse effects can also be categorized by incidence or occurrence over time, or by prevalence indicating which adverse effects tend to be persistent. Within these categories of adverse effects are some which can be characterized as *acute*. This group includes those which are idiosyncratic and may become more severe such as a hypersensitivity reaction with skin rash. A second acute subgroup of adverse effects may be a pharmacodynamic response to medication that improves or disappears with time as tolerance develops. Other adverse effects are chronic or slowly increase with length of exposure to medication. Gum hypertrophy with use of phenytoin is an example of a chronic effect. Adverse effects also includes those related to blood or brain concentration that are reversible by changes in dose. Adverse effects may also be characterized by importance or severity. Idiosyncratic, potentially lethal, hepatotoxicity may be of greater importance than more frequent, but less hazardous problems, such as sedation. Many adverse effects cannot readily be categorized as more or less important or severe because they assume different importance for each individual. To the elderly or institutionalized patient with epilepsy, sexual impotence may be less important than gastrointestinal distress but quite the opposite might be true for a male in his mid 20's. Subjective complaints (e.g., reports of sedation) depend on individual patient or family assessment rather than professional observation and measurement. Nonetheless, it is possible to obtain estimates of subjective problems and record them for analysis. It is also possible to define the magnitude or severity of the complaint with varying degrees of exactness. Unlike laboratory test results that provide specific numbers, problems such as sedation or tremor can be categorized as mild, moderate, and severe, with descriptive definition developed for each category. Scores based on severity can be determined by the clinical judgement of experts.

VA RATING SCALES FOR ADVERSE EFFECTS

The VA group developed a scoring system for the presence and severity of adverse effects. The individual reports were also converted into numerical rating scores based on severity and importance. The format used in the second study was modified from the original scale (Cramer et al., 1983) to measure adverse effects specific for valproate which were not expected in the earlier trial (e.g., weight gain, hair loss). The scoring sheets (Figures 1 and 2) include the recording of specific events as well as the numbers of points assigned to the adverse effect, with the more severe problems receiving a higher score. The design of the scoring was developed so that 50 points were assigned for an adverse effect that was entirely unacceptable for this population group.

Following are brief listings of the types and gradations of specific adverse effects typical of antiepileptic drugs that are included in the VA scales.

Systemic side effects generally include problems with gastrointestinal disorders, such as abdominal distress, nausea and vomiting. The severity of the side effects can be rated as transient or occasional, frequent after medication, or frequent during the day. Haematopoietic system problems include decreased platelet count, reduced white blood cell count, drop in haematocrit or haemoglobin, macrocytic anaemia or reduced red blood cell folate level. Oral and dermatologic problems generally include gum hypertrophy, acne, hirsutism or alopecia of moderate or severe degree. Hypersensitivity reactions include a general maculopapular rash that is transient and clears without stopping treatment, or one that is severe and does not stop, requiring drug discontinuation. Hypersensitivity reactions commonly occur during the first 6 months of treatment, most within the first 2 months (Mattson et al., 1985). Impotence related to drug can involve either libido or decreased potency, either of which can be transient, occasional or continuous and be tolerable or intolerable for the individual. Abnormal liver function tests usually involve a doubling of the normal upper limit for transaminases or rapidly rising levels. Subnormal sodium levels may also occur. Rheumatologic complaints may be associated with barbiturate use (Mattson et al., 1989, Schmidt, 1983). Occasional other adverse effects have been associated with antiepileptic drugs but the above mentioned items cover the preponderance of problems associated with the currently available antiepileptic drugs (Mattson et al, 1986).

VA Systemic Toxicity Rating[a]

Patient's name_____ Study no._____/_____/_____
Form completed by_____ Date _____/_____/_____
                                                                                          (Mo)   (Day)   (Yr)

Rating Period: Baseline 1wk 2wk 1mo 2mo 3mo 4mo 6mo 9mo 12 mo 15mo 18mo 21mo 24mo other___

Instructions: All toxicity is scored relative to normal for this patient before starting this medication.

1. Does patient have any drug-related gastrointestinal
   problems?
   _____ Yes _____ No
   If yes, circle the highest applicable score and enter on
   the appropriate score line. Enter zero on the other two
   score lines.

	Distress	Nausea	Vomiting	Other	SCORE
a. Transient or occasionally after medication	3	5	10	____	____
b. Often after medication	5	10	25	____	____
c. Often during the day	10	25	50	____	____

2. Does the patient have hematopoietic system
   problems?
   _____ Yes _____ No
   If yes, enter a score for each of the following (enter zeros
   if not present):

   a. Reduced platelet count <75,000 (seen on   ___
      more than 1 test
      (Score 25 points if under observation,
      score 50 if drug discontinued)
   b. Reduced WBC <2,000 (1000 granulocytes)   ___
      (seen on more than 1 test) or discontinue drug
      (Score 25 points if under observation,
      score 50 if drug discontinued)
   c. Other hematopoietic problem (describe):
      _____   ___

   d.   Score _____

3. Does patient have a hypersensitivity reaction to the
   study drug (general maculopapular rash)?
   _____ Yes _____ No
   If yes, score one of the following:

   Transient (stopped with treatment)   15
   Severe (did not stop with treatment)   50
   a.   Score _____

4. Does patient have problems with impotence (libido or
   potency)related to drug use?
   _____ Yes _____ No
   If yes, score one of the following:

   Transient, occasional or tolerable   20
   Continuous or intolerable   50
   a.   Score_____

5. Does patient have hyponatremia with serum sodium
   <120 mmol/L ? ____ Yes ____ No
   If yes, score 50.
                   Score _____

6. Does patient have liver disease (related to drug) with
   abnormal liver function tests (SGOT, SGPT repeatedly
   more than twice normal)? (Verify with liver consultant).
   _____ Yes _____ No
   If yes, score 25 if under observation, score 50 if drug
   discontinued.
   a.   Score _____

7. Has patient gained weight because of increased
   appetite related to drug use?
   _____ Yes _____ No
   If yes, score one of the following:

   Weight Gain: Small   (4-6 lbs.)   =   3
                Moderate   (7-12 lbs.) = 10
                Large   (13-18 lbs) = 20
   a.   Score _____

8. Does patient have any changes in hair quantity or
   texture
   since starting drug?
   _____ Yes _____ No
   If yes, score all of the following that apply.

   a. Hair loss:
      Mild: Notice excess hair in comb   5
      Moderate: Visible thinning of hair
      or hair loss in clumps   20
      Severe: Visible alopecia or
      exceedingly bothersome to patient   50

   b. Hair texture or changes other than loss,
      e.g., becoming coarse, fine, curly   5

   c. Hirsutism (excess hair growth):
      Moderate (noticeable on
      face, trunk or limbs)   20
      Severe (excessive and
      bothersome to patient)   50
   d.   Score _____

9. Other (describe):
   _____
                   Score _____

10. **Systemic Toxicity Score (sum of questions 1-9)**
                   Total Score_____

[a] Systemic and Neurotoxicity Rating Scales adapted from scales originally designed for VA Cooperative Study #118 and
described by Cramer et al, Neurology 1983; 33 (Suppl 1):26-37.

Figures 1 and 2. Scoring sheets for VA systemic and neurotoxity ratings.

VA Neurotoxicity Rating[a]

Patient's name_____ Study no._____/_____/_____

Form completed by_____ Date _____/_____/_____

(Mo)   (Day)   (Yr)

Rating Period: Baseline 1wk 2wk 1mo 2mo 3mo 4mo 6mo 9mo 12mo 15mo 18mo 21mo 24mo other ___

Instructions: All toxicity is scored relative to normal for this patient before starting this medication. Do not change drug if toxicity occurs with high serum level; reduce drug dose. Circle all scores that apply and record on score line. Record 0's on score lines if no toxicity is present.

Section A: **Score**

1. **Diplopia**
   a. Intermittent   15
   b. Constant   30 _____

2. **Nystagmus** (not end point):
   a. Horizontal   5
   b. Vertical   10 _____

3. **Dysarthria**
   a. Mild (intermittent slurring)   5
   b. Moderate (constant slurring, no difficulty communicating)   10
   c. Severe (understanding of speech difficult if topic unknown to listener   30 _____

4. **Gait, normal walking:**
   a. Slight ataxia (slowness or unsteady turning)   5
   b. Mild ataxia (veer from side to side, difficulty with tandem gait)   15
   c. Moderate ataxia (unsteady, walks with wide base gait; tendency to fall toward one side or other)   25
   d. Severe gait disturbance (can walk only with assistance, some unsteadiness even when sitting)   50 _____

5. **Rapid Alternating Movements** (hand on knee, flip side to side, grossly clumsy)   15

6. **Tremor** (finger to nose, long reach; eyes open/eyes closed-resting and with arms extended forward):
   [Circle type: Intention - Resting - Postural - None]

   a. Mild (intermittent tremor, not functionally important, noticeable by patient or doctor)   10
   b. Moderate (usually or often evident to patient/doctor on exam: may be embarrassing,
      but no significant compromise: skilled motor acts)   25
   c. Moderately Severe (frequent or constant tremor, compromises to some degree: writing, fine
      motor movement, etc.)   35
   d. Severe (disturbs everyday functioning: eating, writing, working)   50

7. **Enter total for items 1-6** (if more than one score, sum and multiply by 50%; if only one
   score, enter score)

                                                      Section A Score _____

Section B:

8. **Sedation** (level of consciousness):
   a. Lethargic in early A.M. or evening   5
   b. Occasionally sleepy during day   10
   c. Often difficult staying awake   25
   d. Stuporous   50
                                   Score _____

9. **Affect and Mood** (depression tension/agitation; anger/hostility; vigor/excitability;
   fatigue/ apathy; confusion/thought disorder):
   a. Mild (a disturbance is recognized by the patient, but it results in no interference with usual life   5
   b. Moderate (the mood disturbance results in reduced abilities, but only periodically)   15
   c. Severe (continuous or nearly continuous mood disturbance interfering with usual life)   50
                                   Score _____

10. **Cognitive Function** (attention/concentration):
    a. Mild (symptoms recognizable but no interference with usual life)   5
    b. Moderate (interference with some daily activities)   10
    c. Severe (interference with all daily activities)   50

11. **Drug-Related Dizziness/Lightheadiness** (record only highest single score):	Transient or Occasionally After Meds	Often After Meds	Often During Day	Score
a. Mild (symptoms recognizable but no interference with usual life)	3	5	10	
b. Moderate (interference with some daily activities)	5	10	25	
c. Severe (interference with all daily activities)	10	25	50	_____

12. **Drug-Related Headaches** (record only highest single score):				
a. Mild (symptoms recognizable but no interference with usual life	3	5	10	
b. Moderate (interference with some daily activities)	5	10	25	
c. Severe (interference with all daily activities	10	25	30	_____

13. **Other Neurotoxicity** (describe): _____

                                         Score _____

14. **Neurotoxicity Rating Score** (Sum of Questions 7 through 13)

                                         Total Score _____

---

[a] Systemic and Neurotoxicity Rating Scales adapted from scales originally designed for VA Cooperative Study #118 and described by Cramer et al, Neurology 1983; 33 (Suppl 1):26-37.

Much less common but potentially important are drug-related idiosyncratic bone marrow depression, hepatitis, pancreatitis, or vasculitis.

Neurological side effects include disorders of vision such as diplopia and nystagmus. Speech disorders resulting in dysarthria can be mild intermittent slurring, moderate constant slurring without difficulty in communicating, or severe difficulty understanding speech. Motor disorders include abnormal gait during walking with either slight ataxia and slowness or unsteady turning, mild ataxia with veering from side to side and difficulty with tandem gait, or moderate ataxia with unsteadiness, wide based gait, and tendency to fall towards one side or another. Severe gait disturbances allow walking only with assistance and cause poor truncal balance while sitting. Abnormal rapid alternating movements are noted as gross clumsiness. Tremor should be described by type as intention, postural, or resting, and by intensity. Dizziness/lightheadedness and headaches can be noted. The above visual, speech and motor effects often result from the same drug related problem and can be pooled so that scoring the cluster represents a single unit of adverse impact neurologically (Cramer et al., 1983).

Sedation or altered level of consciousness can be noted as lethargy in the early morning or afternoon, occasional sleepiness during the day, frequent difficulty staying awake, or stupor. Changes in affect and mood (including depression, tension/agitation, anger/hostility, vigour/excitability, fatigue/apathy, and confusion/thought disorder) can be reported as a mild disturbance recognized by the patient but resulting in no interference with usual life; moderate mood disturbance resulting in reduced abilities; severe, or nearly continuous mood disturbance interfering with usual life. Cognitive function changes including attention and concentration deficits can be reported as mild with symptoms recognizable but without interference with usual life, moderate interference with some daily activity, or severe interference with all daily activities. These are typical neurotoxicities attributable to the standard antiepileptic drugs (Cramer et al., 1983, Mattson et al., 1986). Some of the newer compounds under development are thought to have psychotropic action that could be exhibited as euphoria or mania.

Neuropsychological effects are measures of subtle neurological problems probably attributable to medication, based on changes in test scores from pre-treatment condition. Neuropsychological test batteries often include a variety of tests selected from measures that can differentiate changes in motor, cognitive, affect, and mood states. Typical motor tests include finger tapping and peg board timed test ratings that evaluate the efficiency and speed of gross and fine motor function. A mixture of hand-eye-learning skills are used in more complex tasks. Cognitive tests include such measures as colour naming, word finding, visual search, paced auditory serial addition tasks, trail making tasks, digit span, digit symbol, critical flicker fusion, reaction time, and other similar tasks. Changes in memory can be assessed using tests such as the Wechsler Memory Score, the Rey-Osterreith Pictorial Memory Test and the Rey Verbal Memory Test. The Profile of Mood States (POMS) measures 6 aspects of mood including tension, depression, anger, vigour, confusion, fatigue. The Minnesota Multiphasic Personality Inventory (MMPI), Washington Psycho-Social Personality Inventory (WPSI) and Wechsler Adult Intelligent Score (WAIS) are not specific measures of drug side effects but are thought to represent more stable measures of general personality and intelligence including verbal and performance abilities. Several test batteries have been shown to detect changes attributable to use of antiepileptic drugs (Dodrill and Troupin, 1975, Novelly et al., 1986, Prevey et al., 1989).

Laboratory tests of blood and urine samples are performed routinely during the assessment of antiepileptic drug efficacy. These general test batteries provide information about the potential systemic changes caused by use of antiepileptic drugs. Commonly, adverse effects caused by these drugs that are noted in laboratory testing are decreased white cell blood count, decreased platelet count, elevated liver function tests including SGOT/SGPT (ASAT/ALAT), decreased sodium, and elevated alkaline phosphatase. Other special tests can be requested if a specific adverse effect is suspected. Test changes often are unassociated with a clinical effect, but may suggest potential problems.

TIMING OF ADVERSE EFFECTS AND EVALUATION

Early Evaluation: Acute side effects usually include the immediate neurological problems that accompany initiation of most central nervous system-active drugs. The typical problems of sedation, dizziness, motor disturbance, and nausea represent problems to which the patients usually become tolerant within days or weeks. Although all antiepileptic drugs may be associated with transient adverse effects, a commonly known example of acute intolerance is seen with initiation of primidone in many patients (Leppik et al., 1984, Mattson et al., 1985, Timberlake et al., 1955). Patients have been known to report immediate dizziness, stupor, ataxia, intense nausea, and projectile vomiting even after a single 125 mg dose (half tablet) of primidone. Those who are able to continue with the slow build up of dosage will develop tolerance, usually within a week or two. However, the intensity and immediacy of these acute problems may lead patients to refuse continuation with that drug. Various idiosyncratic effects caused by all drugs often appear at this time.

Related or independent hepatotoxicity also can be noted during this period with a slow, steady elevation of liver function tests, particularly SGOT (ASAT). Decrease in white blood cell count or platelet count may be noted during the first few months of treatment. Laboratory tests are used to observe changes in any measurement that might be pertinent to drug usage. For example, decreased serum sodium has been associated with use of carbamazepine in a small percentage of patients. The changes can be reversed with decrease or discontinuation of carbamazepine.

During the early assessment of a new compound when dose range is not yet established, patients receiving a high dose can develop acute neurotoxicity that will provide a picture of the type of problems to be expected during "overdose." Mattson et al. (1986) described the time course and type of problems seen acutely with carbamazepine, phenobarbital, phenytoin and primidone.

Later Effects: After the period of acute toxicity and development of tolerance to the drug, or slow dose increase that avoids initial toxicity, patients begin a period of long-term observation. The establishment of a reasonable and optimum dose that prevents seizures but does not cause excessive side effects usually avoids the development of acute systemic and neurotoxicity during this stage of evaluation. However, this is the period where other side effects will appear. Patient often report diminished cognitive abilities and mood changes. Persistent fatigue may be intolerable at doses necessary to control seizures. Problems with libido may not be recognized by the patient as related to the seizure medication, but are known to be associated with barbiturate therapy more than with other drugs.

Chronic Evaluation: Unusual adverse effects can be so rare, and require such a large population base using the drug, that they are not noticed for several years or more after introduction of the compound. Some adverse effects develop only during chronic use and are insidious in onset. Examples of a late developing problem that has been associated with barbiturate usage are connective tissue disorders that can be caused by phenobarbital and primidone (Mattson et al., 1989, Schmidt et al., 1983). Although this adverse effect was noted by French physicians in the 1920's, it is only in the past few years that the issue has been reinvestigated and reported so as to warn physicians to examine patients taking barbituates chronically for Dupuytren's Contractures, palmar nodules, frozen shoulder, Ledderhosen Syndrome, etc. The effect of phenytoin on the cerebellum remains a disputed issue although evidence has long pointed toward cerebellar atrophy after periods of phenytoin intoxication. Affective, cognitive or behavioral effects may be subtle but persistent with long term use.

The clinimetric approach to documentation of the time and type of adverse effects allows for accrual of both a numerator and denominator for estimation of relative risk, as well as incidence and prevalence of the problems.

OCCURRENCE—COLLECTION OF SPECIFIC DATA

Data collected on the VA Systemic and Neurotoxicity Rating Scales were analyzed in two ways. First, any patient who experienced an adverse effect causing unacceptable consequences (e.g., a severe idiosyncratic sensitivity reaction) was dropped from the study and 50 points of toxicity was assigned for that event. Patients were rated for adverse effects at 12 follow up visits, providing a measure of both occurrence and prevalence from acute to chronic therapy. After 12 or 24 months of treatment, all patients in the trial were assessed separately for their toxicity and seizure ratings as well as the combined composite score. Thus, side effects leading to failure were included for all patients entering the study whether they reached 12 or 24 months or not.

These results included scores for patients who were seen at the 12 and 24 month follow-up visits. The purpose of this type of analysis was to determine how patients were doing who had not failed drug. Specifically, drug failure rates could be similar for two treatment programs but the number of side effects chronically experienced might be higher for one drug than another. In the initial study, carbamazepine and phenytoin had lower (better) scores but the differences did not reach statistical significance. In the second VA study, carbamazepine and valproate were compared both for incidence of adverse effects as well as prevalence at a given point in time. Valproate caused significantly more tremor, hair change, and large weight gain than carbamazepine, whereas carbamazepine caused more hypersensitivity reactions.

SEVERITY OF ADVERSE EFFECTS

The severity of specific adverse effects (e.g., tremor, gastrointestinal disturbance, headache, lightheadedness) not only was noted for presence or absence, but also was characterized by degree of severity. Specific numbers of adverse effect points were assigned for the score to be used in the rating scale but also provided groups allowing enumeration of adverse effects. The quantification of adverse effects is well illustrated by the assessment of recurring tremor. Tremor was found significantly more frequent with use of valproate than carbamazepine. The characterization of tremor severity made it possible to demonstrate that mild and moderate tremor was much more common with use of valproate than for carbamazepine. However, the number of patients who experienced a clinically severe adverse effect of any type was relatively small.

Following are Tables 1 and 2, listing the mean neurotoxicity scores and mean composite scores for patients taking carbamazepine and valproate (in the second VA study). Higher systemic toxicity scores (not shown) for patients taking valproate probably reflect weight gain and hair change. Higher neurotoxicity scores for patients taking valproate probably reflect tremor.

SHORTCOMINGS

The rating scales allow assignment of numerical scores that can be combined to give an overall score or rating of adverse effects as a clinical phenomenon. In addition to providing quantification of outcomes, ratings allow comparison of clinical outcome for patients treated with various regimens by characteristics other than seizure control. The risk exists that a single item in a rating scale may be sufficiently powerful to affect the outcome of all adverse effects combined. For example, the neurotoxicity rating comparing valproate with carbamazepine resulted in scores that were significantly different although only one measure of neurotoxicity (e.g., tremor) was more frequent with use of valproate

Table 1. Mean neurotoxicity scores (maximum score = 50)

RATING	N	MEAN CBZ	SD	N	MEAN VPA	SD
1 week	193	5.1	9	196	4.0	8
1 mo	202	4.9	8	207	3.7	6
3 mo	163	5.2	10	176	4.8	9
6 mo	147	3.9	8	164	5.9	9
12 mo	127	2.8	6	136	7.3	10
18 mo	96	3.3	6	102	5.1	8
24 mo	89	2.5	6	88	5.0	8

Table 2. Composite scores of seizures and toxicity ratings[a]

SEIZURE GROUP	CBZ	VPA	P
Gen'l Tonic-Clonic			
12 mo	9.4	13.8	0.39
24 mo	6.1	10.7	0.37
Complex Partial			
12 mo	6.8	16.0	<0.0001
24 mo	8.2	13.6	0.14
Both Groups			
12 mo	8.3	14.8	0.002
24 mo	7.0	11.9	0.11

[a]The lower the score, the better the outcome

than carbamazepine. Such a measurement can mislead a reader to conclude that all aspects of neurotoxicity (instead of a single type) were involved in the less favourable neurotoxicity score. A simple listing of the incidence or prevalence, supplemented by severity of adverse effect, is more informative for such documentation.

Important differences may also be lost by combining scores. Thus, weight gain was significantly more common with valproate use, whereas idiosyncratic rash was more frequent with carbamazepine. Combining the scores suggests that the two drugs did not differ in overall systemic toxicity and fails to clearly identify important selective differences. Timing of analyses may also effect ratings. Systemic toxicity such as weight gain or hair change will persist with chronic use of valproate, whereas serious carbamazepine hypersensitive reactions will cause drug failure. Analyses of systemic toxicity scores found at 12 months may suggest that carbamazepine has less toxicity than valproate because patients with early, severe adverse experiences were removed from the trial.

ALTERNATIVE MEASURES

Many clinical trials have incorporated some elements of graded severity or importance although adverse effect rating systems have not been used. A major methodologic difference between the recording of adverse events in the VA study and some other systems is the means of detecting and recording these events. The VA study elicited reporting of adverse events while many other groups use spontaneous reports of complaints or descriptions from the patient or family. In the VA studies, every patient was asked on every visit about the presence of every potential adverse effect noted on the forms, and the frequency and severity was also recorded. The advantage of spontaneous reporting of adverse effects is that fewer trivial and non-drug-related items are reported, and this corresponds more closely to usual clinical practice. The disadvantage of such an approach is underreporting of adverse effects associated with treatment. Some patients may be unaware of uncommon drug effects such as hair thinning and might fail to report it because they assumed the problem was related to some other factor. Some uncertainty exists as to how many patients not only experienced a problem (numerator) but also how many patients were assessed for a specific problem (denominator). By specifically asking or examining for certain adverse effects in a structured format, both a numerator and denominator are obtained with much more precision to determine the number and percent of individuals affected by an adverse effect. Such a measure, however, not only maximizes reporting but may include many unwanted symptoms or abnormalities unrelated to either the antiepileptic drug use or the epilepsy. For example, depression or other psychological disturbances may be entirely related to psychosocial events independent of the medical problem. Efforts can be made by the examiner to differentiate clearly non-drug or non-disease related events but attribution may be difficult at times.

USE OF ADVERSE EFFECT RATINGS FOR OVERALL OUTCOME

Rating scores provide important information about various aspects of adverse effects associated with use of antiepileptic drugs. This in itself is important clinical information but it also may be combined with seizure efficacy measures to provide an overall assessment. Ultimately, a measure of a drug's usefulness can best be found in the therapeutic index or ratio of seizure efficacy and adverse effects. A modestly effective drug may be more desirable for some patients if adverse effects are minimal compared to a highly potent antiepileptic drug which carries more frequent or severe adverse effects. Such a determination will depend on what is of greatest importance to the individual patient. A global assessment is one means of gaining an overall determination of successful treatment. Such an assessment often incorporates seizure control, adverse effects, subjective feelings of satisfaction, and other psychosocial aspects. A composite score is a quantitative expression of some of these issues. In the VA study, the seizure and adverse effect scores were totalled to give a composite score. Excellent seizure control but with moderate adverse effects might yield a moderate score. If dosage were lowered in the same individual to relieve some adverse effects, seizure score might increase so that the composite score would remain approximately the same. Thus, an overall estimate of outcome with use of this drug can be achieved. Wijsman et al (1991) have recently carried out both retrospective and prospective studies using a modification of this scoring system and found good interrater reliability as well as a positive correlation between frequency of return visits and overall composite score.

SUMMARY AND CONCLUSIONS

Multiple measures of adverse effects of antiepileptic drugs, other than clinical impressions or nominal descriptions are important to gain an appreciation of the frequency, severity, and type of effects as well as their relationship to seizure control. A specific rating method was used in two multicentre VA Cooperative Studies which enroled 1,102 patients with symptomatic, localization-related epilepsy. These methods help provide a quantitative tool of assessment for the effects of antiepileptic drugs. The adverse effect scores are also valuable when combined with those of seizure rating to produce a composite number that provides a relative estimate of overall successful outcome with use of various drugs. It is recognized that a number of limitations and pitfalls exist in use of such a measurement system and opportunities exist for modification or refinement by other groups especially when the scales are used for different purposes. The rating scale for adverse events did not replace traditional recording methods, but were used as a supplementary tool. Our experience indicates that quantification of clinical events (clinimetrics) is applicable and valuable in the assessment of antiepileptic drug adverse effects.

REFERENCES

Bourgeois B, Beaumanoir A, Blajev B, et al. Monotherapy with valproate in primary generalized epilepsies. Epilepsia 1987; 28 sup2:S8–S11.

Cramer JA, Smith DB, Mattson RH, et al. A method of quantification for the evaluation of antiepileptic drug therapy. Neurology 1983; 33:26–37.

Dodrill CB, Troupin AS. Effects of repeated administrations of a comprehensive neuropsychological battery among chronic epileptics. J Nerv Ment Dis 1975; 3:185–190.

Feinstein AR. Clinimetrics. New Haven: Yale University Press, 1987.

Heller AJ, Chesterman P, Elwes RDC, et al. Monotherapy for newly diagnosed epilepsy: A comparative trial and prognostic evaluation. Epilepsia 1989; 30:648.

Leppik IE, Cloyd JC, Miller K. Development of tolerance to the side effects of primidone. Ther Drug Monit 1984; 6:189–191.

Mattson RH. Selection of antiepileptic drug therapy. In: Levy R, et al., eds, Antiepileptic Drugs, Third Edition. New York: Raven Press, 1989:103–115.

Mattson RH, Cramer JA. Assessment of antiepileptic drug efficacy and toxicity. In: Shorvon SD, Birdwood GFB, eds. Rational approaches to anticonvulsant drug therapy. Berne: Hans Huber publishers, 1984:22–27.

Mattson RH, Cramer JA, Collins JF, et al. Comparison of carbamazepine, phenobarbital, phenytoin, and primidone in partial and secondary generalized tonic-clonic seizures. N Engl J Med 1985; 313:145–151.

Mattson RH, Cramer JA, Collins JF, and the VA Epilepsy Cooperative Study Group. Early tolerance to antiepileptic drug side effects: A controlled trial of 247 patients. In: Frey H-H et al, ed. Tolerance to Beneficial and/or Adverse Effects of Antiepileptic Drugs. New York: Raven Press, 1986:149–156.

Mattson RH, Cramer JA, McCutchen CB, and the VA Epilepsy Cooperative Study Group. Barbiturate related connective tissue disorders. Arch Int Med 1989; 149:911–914.

Mattson RH, Cramer JA, Collins JF, and the VA Epilepsy Cooperative Study No. 264 Group. A comparison of valproate with carbamazepine for the treatment of partial seizures and secondarily generalized tonic-clonic seizures in adults. N Engl J Med 1992; 327:765–777.

Novelly RA, Schwartz MM, Mattson RH, Cramer JA. Behavioral toxicity associated with antiepileptic drugs. Epilepsia 1986; 27:331–340.

Prevey ML, Mattson RH, Cramer JA. Improvement in cognitive functioning and mood state after conversion to valproate monotherapy. Neurology 1989; 39:1640–1641.

Schmidt D. Connective tissue disorders induced by antiepileptic drugs. In: Oxley J, et al, eds. Antiepileptic Drug Therapy: Chronic Toxicity of Antiepileptic Drugs. New York: Raven Press, 1983:115–124.

Timberlake WH, Abbott JA, Schwab RS. An effective anticonvulsant with initial problems of adjustment. N Engl J Med 1955; 7:252–304.

Wijsman DJP, Hekster YA, Renier WO, Meinardi H. Clinimetrics and epilepsy care. Pharm Weekbl [sci] 1991; 13:182–188.

CONVENTIONAL AND CLINIMETRIC APPROACHES TO INDIVIDUALIZATION OF ANTIEPILEPTIC DRUG THERAPY

John S. Duncan M.A., D.M., M.R.C.P.

Epilepsy Research Group
Institute of Neurology
National Hospital for Neurology and Neurosurgery
Queen Square, London WC1N 3BG, United Kingdom

and

Chalfont Centre for Epilepsy
Buckinghamshire, United Kingdom

INTRODUCTION

The goal of the physician treating an individual patient with epilepsy is to help them to achieve the best quality of life possible, by careful tailoring of their antiepileptic drug (AED) treatment and attention to the wider implications of epilepsy.

The conventional approach to the drug treatment of epilepsy has been to balance the numbers of seizures of different types reported by the patient against overt side-effects of AEDs. The current issue is whether AED treatment may be improved by adoption of a clinimetric approach.

Seizures, side-effects of AEDs and the overall well-being of a patient need to be considered when advising patients about their drug treatment. Essentially, these items form the physical and psychological domains of a proposed epilepsy quality of life scale (Table 1) (Duncan 1990; Vickrey et al. 1993). Performance in the social and occupational domains will largely depend on the physical and psychological domains and also on external environmental and socio-economic factors, some of which are beyond medical intervention, such as finance, family, friends and housing.

There are important practical limitations to the clinimetric approach and it is necessary to distinguish research questions from clinical management issues. When considering a clinimetric approach an important point is the great heterogeneity between patients in

Quantitative Assessment in Epilepsy Care, Edited by H. Meinardi et al.
Plenum Press, New York, 1993

137

Table 1. Factors affecting quality of life in epilepsy

Domain	Items
Physical	• Frequency and severity of seizures • Sedation • Impairment of function • Mobility • Sexual functioning
Psychological	• Depression • Anxiety • Adjustment to illness • Cognitive function and memory
Social	• Personal relationships • Ability to enjoy social and leisure activity
Occupational	• Ability to cope with household duties and day to day life, independently • Ability to obtain and retain employment

terms of age, occupation, intellect and cognition, neurological or psychiatric deficit, seizure frequency and severity, personality and outlook on life.

In a research protocol it is necessary to know what questions are being asked, by whom they are being asked and for what purpose, before designing a clinimetric scale. Principal issues in a short term study are seizure frequency and severity, side-effects from AEDs and some measure of mood and patient satisfaction. In longer term assessments, there may be greater emphasis on whether the patient's epilepsy is in remission or not, whether there are any side-effects from medication or not, and a measure of the patient's perceived quality of life.

It is not likely to prove feasible or useful to try to develop a single, all purpose scale for measuring quality of life in patients with epilepsy, but more profitable to employ scales that are designed to answer specific questions. Further potential concerns about the clinimetric approach are that assigning numerical scores implies a scientific process and, if these are not validated, may generate pseudoscience and a plethora of data that could be abused, for example by interested parties who may wish to demonstrate that one AED is superior to another.

In clinical practice a clinimetric approach to the medical treatment of patients with epilepsy has the attraction of appearing to offer rational treatment strategies for difficult clinical circumstances. Whilst this may be the case, a reservation about the widespread adoption of the clinimetric approach into clinical practice is that an excessive reliance on numbers may be to the detriment of clinical competence in a routine setting. By analogy, serum AED concentration data are often abused by naive physicians, and not infrequently lead to inappropriate treatment of the numerical data rather than careful consideration of the individual patient.

COMPOSITE CLINICAL SCORES

There have already been attempts to adopt a clinimetric approach and to derive an overall measure of efficacy of AED treatment and of side-effects. Cramer et al. (1983) described a composite scoring system for quantifying the beneficial and adverse effects of AEDs being evaluated in the Veterans' Administration multi-centre studies. A key feature of this system is that the scores of all the factors are summed to yield a single number. This is superficially attractive, but amalgamates very different data that are not readily equatable e.g. number of complex partial seizures in a week, platelet count, nausea and coordination. This approach does not allow for differences in what matters to patients: intermittent diplopia or a white cell count of 2.8×10^9/litre may not trouble one man at all, so long as his seizures are controlled. As a result this scale is not likely to be useful when individualizing patients' drug treatment. Nevertheless, this scale does provide a handle by which the investigator or physician may get some idea as to whether the treatment is going well, is mediocre, or not satisfactory; and may also help to ensure a degree of consistency in clinical management between different sites in a multi-centre study.

Wijsman et al. (1991) adapted the Veterans' Administration scale and measured seizure activity, systemic and neurological toxicity in patients with chronic epilepsy who were attending an epilepsy clinic. Thirteen percent of patients were seizure free, and only 10% had no impairment (i.e. no seizures and no side-effects of medication), reflecting the nature of the population selected for the study. Systemic toxicity was recorded in 7% and neurotoxicity in 20%. In 80% of patients the composite score was less than 50, thought to represent a satisfactory result. A reservation about these data is the arbitrary nature of the cut off, and the fact that scores appear to reflect professional opinion and not necessarily what matters to individual patients. For example, the occurrence of two complex partial seizures per week gave rise to a lower score than would the occurrence of two generalized tonic clonic seizures in a year. For some patients, the latter would be the preferable situation, particularly if the complex partial seizures were associated with prolonged and socially disabling automatisms. This illustrates the limitations of trying to use a clinimetric approach to guide treatment. The study, however, has shown that such a scale may be implemented in an epilepsy clinic without undue difficulty and gave an overview of the health of the patients attending, and of the prevalence of adverse effects.

Assessment of Seizure Frequency and Severity

The counting of the numbers of different types of seizures occurring in a unit time is an established clinimetric technique for measuring drug efficacy and for guiding treatment. Recent variations on this theme have been advocated, such as time taken for the occurrence of a predetermined number of seizures, and the number of seizure free days in a unit time (Shofer and Temkin 1986). It is not yet clear how useful these measures may be when optimizing individual patient's AED treatment in clinical practice. With prospective recording in diaries, this data is relatively easy to collect and reliable for tonic-clonic and clear cut complex partial seizures, although quantification of absences and simple partial seizures is much less likely to be accurate.

The severity of seizures is an important aspect of epilepsy that matters to patients and their careers. This has been recognized for many years (Gruber et al. 1957; Cereghino et al. 1974), but scores of the relative severity of different seizure types have been arbitrary. Appropriate methodology for measuring this parameter has been developed only recently, beginning with the Veterans' Administration Cooperative Studies (Cramer et al. 1983). In the last two years there have been further studies in the UK to quantify seizure severity, at Liverpool (Baker et al. 1991) and at the Chalfont Centre for Epilepsy (Duncan and Sander 1991).

The Chalfont Seizure Severity Scale comprises 11 factors that were commonly felt, by patients and their relatives, to be disruptive and disturbing features of seizures. The factors were loss of awareness, presence or absence of a warning, dropping of a held object, fall to the ground, injury, incontinence, automatisms, convulsion, duration of seizure, time taken to return to normal and diurnal pattern. In common with other clinical epileptological data, seizure severity scores depend on a reliable history being available from the patient and a witness to the seizures.

The Chalfont scale was designed to provide an objective measure of the severity of seizures, concentrating on those aspects that cause disturbance to patients and their relatives and, deliberately, was intended not to be constrained by the International Classification of Seizures. It was not intended to be a measure of the impact of epilepsy on the life of an individual, which will depend on several other factors—both internal and external. Seizure severity data is independent of seizure frequency and may be collected for each type of seizure. A possible development, which may be a useful measure of the activity of epilepsy and of the efficacy of AEDs, but which has not been validated, would be to multiply seizure frequency and severity for each type of seizure experienced and then to sum the totals, to give an overall 'Seizure Activity Score'.

The seizure severity scale recently devised in Liverpool (Baker et al. 1991) comprises 16 items (6 questions relating to patients' perception of control and 10 to ictal and post-ictal phenomena). Each item could be rated on a 4-point scale, so that the minimum possible score for a seizure type would be 16, and the maximum score 64. This scale was recently used to demonstrate a reduction in seizure severity in some patients who participated in an add-on study of lamotrigine (Smith et al. 1991).

Measurement of seizure severity is feasible, although there is not yet a consensus on the best techniques to employ. It is likely that seizure severity scores will be useful as a measure of AED efficacy in new drug evaluations. In clinical practice, measurement of seizure severity may, along with seizure frequency, be a useful parameter for determining the effects of AEDs and aid changes of treatment towards optimal therapy.

Evaluation of Drug Side-effects

The conventional approach has been to ask about side-effects and if they are troublesome to reduce the dose, or change drug, and reach a compromise between seizure control and patient perceived degree of side-effects.

Key questions are:

(1) Can decisions regarding the antiepileptic drug treatment of individual patients be improved upon by quantifying side-effects?

(2) Does it make sense to try to summate a score for seizures and a score for side-effects and to go for optimization of a composite score.

Quantification of side-effects of AEDs, in both the short term and the long term, is an important part of research protocols. In clinical practice, however, the occurrence of side-effects in the short term and in the longer term, needs to be weighed against the beneficial effects of a drug, but this is an individual decision for a patient with some guidance from the physician and is not likely to be influenced by a numerical score. The use of a composite score in clinical practice is not likely to be beneficial, because of patient variability in terms of epilepsy, concomitant problems and their own judgement of what side-effects are worth tolerating to obtain better suppression of seizures.

PROPOSAL

It may be that a simple patient-based overall measure of satisfaction with their AED treatment could be of some benefit when trying to individualize AED therapy to the optimal for each patient. This could take the form of Visual Analogue Scales, with questions such as:

How satisfied are you with your antiepileptic drug treatment?

Not at all satisfied   Totally satisfied
1_____5

The control of your seizures is:

Totally unsatisfactory   Completely satisfactory
1_____5

Side-effects of your medication are:

Intolerable   None at all
1_____5

CONCLUSIONS

(1) In clinical epilepsy practice, the aim of therapy is:
  • No seizures, minimum number of less severe seizures.
  • A simple AED regimen, with 1–2 doses per day.
  • No adverse drug effects.
  • Satisfied, well adjusted, independent and fully functioning patients.

(2) In research protocols, it is useful to measure seizure frequency, severity and side-effects of AEDs.

(3) Measurement scales should be tailored to the question being asked, rather than trying to use a universal scale, which is likely to become cumbersome and insensitive.

(4) The combination of unrelated variables, e.g. seizure numbers and side-effects, may be useful for helping to ensure consistent treatment policies in multicentre studies but carries the potential risk of generating spurious and misleading data.

(5) In the treatment of individual patients, recording of seizure frequency and severity is important, as is the occurrence of side-effects. Therapy will probably be best individualized for each patient by recognizing what symptoms and signs are drug side-effects and by the patient and physician agreeing what side-effects, if any, are an acceptable price to pay for varying degrees of seizure control.

REFERENCES

Baker GA, Smith DF, Dewey M, Morrow J, Crawford PM, Chadwick DW. The development of a seizure severity scale as an outcome measure in epilepsy. Epilepsy Res 1991; 8: 245–251.

Cereghino JJ, Brock JT, Van Meter JC et al. Evaluation of albutoin as an antiepileptic drug. Clin Pharmacol Ther 1974; 15: 406–416.

Cramer JA, Smith DB, Mattson RH et al. A method of quantification for the evaluation of antiepileptic drug therapy. Neurology 1983; 33 (suppl 1): 26–37.

Duncan JS. Medical factors affecting quality of life in patients with epilepsy. In: Chadwick DW., ed. Quality of life and quality of care in epilepsy. Royal Society of Medicine Round Table Series 1990; 23: 80–87.

Duncan JS, Sander JWAS. The Chalfont seizure severity scale. J Neurol Neurosurg Psychiat 1991; 54: 873–876.

Gruber CM, Mosier JM, Grant P. Objective comparison of primidone and phenobarbitone in epileptics. J Pharmacol Exp Ther 1957; 120: 184–187.

Shofer JB, Temkin NR. Comparison of alternative outcome measures for antiepileptic drug trials. Arch Neurol 1986; 43: 877–881.

Smith D, Baker GA, Dewey M, Chadwick DW. Seizure severity scale as an outcome measure in a double-blind cross-over trial of lamotrigine as add-on therapy in patients with refractory epilepsy. Epilepsia 1991; 32 (suppl 1): 95.

Vickrey BG, Hays RD, Herman B, Batzel L. Quality of life outcomes. In: Engel J, Jr., ed. Surgical treatment of the epilepsies, 2nd edition, Raven Press, New York, 1993.

Wijsman DJP, Hekster YA, Keyser A, Renier WO, Meinardi H. Clinimetrics and epilepsy care. Pharmaceutisch Weekblad Scientific edition 1991; 13: 182–188.

PSYCHOSOCIAL CONSEQUENCES OF EPILEPSY

Jan Vermeulen, D.Psychol.[1] and Raphael Canger, M.D., Ph.D.[2]

[1]Instituut voor Epilepsiebestrijding
Heemstede, The Netherlands

[2]Regional Epilepsy Centre
S. Paolo Hospital
and University of Milan Medical School
Milan, Italy

INTRODUCTION

There is abundant evidence that people with epilepsy, as a group, have more psychological and social problems than normal people. In some individuals such problems may be more debilitating than the seizures themselves. The topics reviewed here represent problem areas on which considerable debate has centred. They are: developmental problems, personality traits, aggression, sexual dysfunction, psychiatric illness and general socioeconomic status in epilepsy.

An examination of the psychosocial ramifications of epilepsy would be incomplete without consideration of the methodological problems involved, but an extended discussion would be beyond the scope of this paper (for a detailed review see Hermann & Whitman, 1984). It is important to note, however, that considerable methodological difficulties obscure an accurate assessment of the psychosocial impact of epilepsy. Methodological issues include sample selection effects and the choice of adequate control groups, controversies regarding measures of personality and psychopathology, the possible influence of various confounding variables such as the use of antiepileptic medication, the effects of economic and social stresses associated with chronic disorders in general. Due to such methodological problems it is rarely clear exactly who or what is being evaluated, and strong conclusions can generally not be made.

Having epilepsy, particularly in the form of intractable seizures, has a number of consequences that often seem severe enough to explain anything from mild depression to paranoid delusions as an understandable psychological reaction to the stresses induced by living with the disorder and its consequences. It would be surprising if factors such as the

Quantitative Assessment in Epilepsy Care, Edited by H. Meinardi et al.
Plenum Press, New York, 1993

145

unpredictable and traumatic nature of the seizures, the ignorance and stigma still associated with epilepsy, or the limitations of activities and aspirations resulting from having a chronic disease, did not have a considerable influence on an individual's psychological status.

There is fairly general agreement, however, that various emotional and personality correlates of epilepsy represent more than simply an understandable psychological reaction to the emotional trauma of physical, social, or cognitive disability. That is, neurophysiological-neurochemical mechanisms, particularly those reflecting limbic system dysfunction, may be involved as well. Because the temporal lobe, and the limbic structures contained within it, are known to be important in the mediation of emotional, sexual and social behaviour in animals, one might expect that people with epilepsy originating in the temporal lobe are at special risk for developing emotional and social difficulties, psychiatric disorders and personality problems. Indeed, Gibbs and Stamps (1953), observing a high incidence of emotional disorders in persons with psychomotor epilepsy, suggested that psychological factors are less important determinants of these disorders than the location of the epileptogenic focus. A very large body of literature now exists concerning the etiological importance of temporal lobe dysfunction in the psychological and social difficulties of people with epilepsy.

Both approaches to psychosocial problems in epilepsy will be considered here. Limbic system dysfunction may indeed be an important factor predisposing people with epilepsy to emotional and behavioral disorders, but in individual cases the form and severity of such disorders presumably depends on an interaction with other factors, including an individual's past experience and his current psychological and social status (Hermann et al., 1982).

DEVELOPMENTAL ASPECTS

Epilepsy with onset in early childhood may have adverse effects on parental and peer group attitudes and the learning of social and academic skills. Restrictions on the individual's activities and lifestyle due to the epilepsy may interfere with personality maturation and contribute to psychosocial difficulties later in life (Fenton, 1981). Parents may worry about the seizures, the side effects of antiepileptic medication or possible future social handicaps (West, 1979; Ward & Bower, 1978). Parents tend to have differential expectations of their children with epilepsy relative to their healthy children, such as more emotional problems, poorer concentration, lower academic achievement and fewer employment opportunities (Long and Moore, 1979). Because of such special concerns and expectations parents may behave differently toward their children with epilepsy. However, there is considerable variation among parents and other members of the family in their reactions to a child with epilepsy, which may range from overprotection to rejection and scapegoating. Various developmental problems may occur due to such extreme reactions, e.g. low self-esteem, lack of social skills (Fenton, 1981), feelings of guilt or the adoption of a sick role (Lechtenberg, 1984), which may have significant effects in adult life. While clinical experience suggests that parental attitudes and expectations are important to an individual's psychosocial development, systematic empirical investigations of the impact of such factors are still rare. The development of objective scales that capture parental attitudes and expectations would greatly contribute to our understanding of this problem area.

Children with epilepsy, as a group, also run a greater risk for developing learning problems. However, "learning problems" has been used as a rather ill-defined category and there is no uniformity in assessment methods. Consequently, prevalence estimates of learning problems in children with epilepsy vary widely, percentages mentioned in the literature ranging from 5 to 50% (Thompson, 1987). Approximately one third receive some form of special educational support (Aldenkamp, 1983; Thompson, 1987). Academic underachievement in children with epilepsy relative to their own abilities has been signalled by several authors (Aldenkamp, 1983; Seidenberg et al., 1986). Parental attitudes and behaviour may reasonably be expected to influence the child's learning behaviour. However, specific cognitive deficits may be responsibly for learning problems and underachievement as well. Slowing on speeded tasks involving complex information processing and quick decision making, attention and concentration difficulties are well established phenomena in epilepsy (Aldenkamp et al., 1990; Alpherts & Aldenkamp, 1990). Factors such as the localisation of the epileptogenic focus, the seizure activity and the central side effects of antiepileptic medication may underlie such cognitive deficits and thus interfere with learning processes.

Disappointing school achievement, regardless of its origin, may have a considerable impact on the self-perception of the child with epilepsy, and may lead to reduced employment choices and earning potential as an adult.

PERSONALITY

The existence of a global "epileptic personality," a particular constellation of unusual personality and behavioral characteristics shared by patients with epilepsy as a group, is debated, and this concept may well represent another example of the prejudices that surround epilepsy. Traits that have traditionally been associated with epilepsy include excessive religiosity, mental slowness, viscosity, circumstantiality, irritability, impulsivity and mood fluctuations. The question as to whether there is a cluster of traits specifically associated with temporal lobe epilepsy (Bear, 1979; Waxman & Geschwind, 1975) is still open. While people with temporal lobe epilepsy tend to have more behavioral problems than normal controls, it is uncertain whether they also show more disturbances than other subjects with chronic brain-related disorders. Also, comparisons of subjects having temporal lobe epilepsy with those having other seizure types with little or no involvement of limbic structures generally do not reveal significant personality differences (Hermann & Whitman, 1984; Strauss, 1989). Such differences either do not exist or they are elusive to detection with current evaluation procedures (e.g. the MMPI), a possibility that has prompted some investigators (e.g. Bear and Fedio, 1977) to devise new rating scales specifically intended to capture traits thought to be specific for temporal lobe epilepsy. However, the merits of such special measures remain unclear. Before they can be used with any confidence in the study of personality in epilepsy, the standard psychometric procedures should be applied such as establishing their reliability and exploring their correlations with other variables of interest e.g. intelligence and other personality measures of demonstrated reliability and validity.

AGGRESSIVE AND SEXUAL BEHAVIOUR

Despite anecdotal reports in the medico-legal literature, suggesting that violent events might be due to epilepsy, the weight of the evidence does not support such allegations (Treiman, 1986; Treiman & Delgado-Escueta, 1983). It is extremely unusual for patients with epilepsy to behave aggressively during a seizure. Also, limbic stimulation rarely evokes anger or aggression. Aggressive behaviour sometimes occurs as a postictal phenomenon because the patient is restrained in an attempt to protect him. Aggressive behaviour during seizures, if it occurs at all, is typically simple, stereotyped, unsustained, unplanned and never supported by a consecutive series of purposeful acts, is not premeditated and does not occur in response to preictal provocation (Strauss, 1989). It is thus not likely that a coordinated act of violence or aggression against others could occur as part of a seizure.

Another issue is whether people with epilepsy, particularly temporal lobe epilepsy, are more irritable, hostile or violent, features that have long been considered part of the "epileptic personality," during the interictal period relative to e.g. healthy controls or other subjects with a chronic illness. Surveys of hospital based clinics generally fail to reveal increased aggression in people with epilepsy in general and temporal lobe epilepsy in particular. Surveys of penal institutions (where more violence-prone individuals might be found) in the U.S. and England have revealed an increased prevalence of epilepsy relative to the general population. However, prisoners with epilepsy did not commit more serious crimes or more crimes of violence compared to their non-epileptic counterparts. Prisoners with temporal lobe epilepsy did not commit more violent crimes than those having other seizure types (Hermann and Whitman, 1984).

Sexual behaviour during seizures may consist of somatosensory sensations in the genitalia, probably due to discharges from the post central gyrus, that may be unpleasant or emotionally neutral. Sexual automatisms i.e. mannerisms such as exhibitionism and other sexual activities that may be related to frontal seizure origin, and erotic feelings that typically indicate the involvement of temporal-limbic structures, may also occur (Strauss,1989).

Few methodologically sound studies have been carried out on interictal sexual function in people with epilepsy. However, the existing data suggest that sexual dysfunction is not uncommon in epilepsy, particularly temporal lobe epilepsy. Hyposexuality, usually in the form of a global loss of performance as well as interest in sex, is the most prominent abnormality, and appears to be specifically associated with temporal lobe epilepsy. However, the presence of temporal lobe epilepsy is presumably only one of the several factors that may contribute to sexual dysfunction in epilepsy. The individual's overall mental health is an important consideration, depressed or anxious subjects may have little interest in sex. The chronic use of antiepileptic drugs may produce alterations in sex hormone levels and thus affect sexual functioning. People with epilepsy may have limited opportunities for social and thus sexual contacts because they are institutionalized or otherwise socially isolated (Hermann & Whitman, 1984; Strauss, 1989).

AFFECT

Fear is the ictal affect most commonly reported as part of a seizure, and is experienced by about 3% of patients with epilepsy. It may also be produced by experimental electrical stimulation of limbic structures, especially the amygdala. Ictal fear typically occurs with temporal lobe seizures, about 20% of subjects with such seizures reporting ictal fear, which differs from the normal state in that it arises suddenly out of context and is undirected. Its duration varies from seconds to minutes, its intensity ranges from mild anxiety to overwhelming terror. Ictal depression, manifested in feelings of sadness, futility and such, and unmotivated by the context, may occur as an aura, during the seizure, or as a sequel to the seizure. Ictal depression is fairly uncommon, occurring in about 1% of the patients with epilepsy, and is associated with temporal-limbic discharges. The duration of the depression may be brief, lasting for minutes, but unlike other ictal emotions the mood may persist for days after the attack. Pleasurable emotions such as feelings of euphoria or gladness can also occur as part of an ictal event, but are extremely rare (see Strauss, 1989 for a review of the literature on ictal affect).

The major interictal affective disorders in epilepsy are depression and anxiety, though their exact prevalence is not known, and relevant studies are too few to establish a specific association with temporal lobe epilepsy (Hermann & Whitman, 1984) or clarify the underlying mechanisms. Psychosocially oriented explanations have emphasized the various psychological and social stresses associated with having seizures. Seizures are essentially unpredictable traumatic events over which the individual has little or no control. The nature of epilepsy thus may be conducive to learned helplessness (Seligman (1975), and it has been suggested that this may be one way of understanding some of the interictal behavioral concomitants of epilepsy, particularly the apparent high rates of anxiety and depression (Hermann, 1979). Medical misinformation, fear of seizures and fear of death from seizures is widespread among patients, and this may affect behaviour in adverse ways. Patients have many concerns about what they think are the potentially destructive effects of epilepsy, i.e. progressive brain damage, mental deterioration, mental illness, loss of intelligence. A common approach to dealing with such fears and concerns is social and emotional withdrawal. Depression and anxiety in epilepsy may in part be due to such mechanisms (Mittan & Locke, 1982). Various measures of depression and anxiety are readily available, e.g. the Depression scale of the MMPI or the Hamilton scale.

PSYCHOPATHOLOGY

A wide variety of simple and complex sensory and perceptual experiences as well as alterations in cognitive and emotional states, can be elicited by temporal lobe seizures. Many of the phenomena experienced during partial complex seizures can also occur in psychiatric illness, e.g. hallucinations and illusions, feelings of depersonalization or forced thinking. When occurring as ictal events they have a sudden onset and rapid resolution, and the attacks have a stereotyped quality.

There is little doubt that overall rates of interictal psychopathology of any type are elevated in epilepsy relative to healthy controls. This increased tendency toward psychopathology appears to be due to the presence of a chronic disorder rather than the epilepsy in itself. Comparisons to patients with other chronic disorders generally fail to reveal increased overall psychopathology rates in epilepsy.

There is evidence that psychopathology when present in epilepsy is more likely to manifest itself as psychosis, particularly schizophrenia-like and paranoid states, than in chronically ill controls (Whitman et al., 1984). This finding might account for the observed overrepresentation of patients with epilepsy in psychiatric hospitals and the increased rates of previous psychiatric hospitalizations in epilepsy, as patients with psychotic disorders are more likely to receive treatment in inpatient psychiatric settings (Hermann & Whitman, 1984). However, there are as yet no population based studies on the prevalence of psychosis in epilepsy that might resolve the question whether or not the combination of epilepsy and psychosis is coincidental. The Diagnostic and Statistical Manual offers a suitable framework for classifying the presenting symptomatology in future investigations of this issue.

The nature of the association (if any) between psychosis and epilepsy is controversial. Data pertaining to a possible link between psychosis and temporal lobe epilepsy and other specific determining factors are contradictory. Despite such uncertainties various neurophysiological and biochemical explanations for a causal link between epilepsy and psychosis have been advanced (see e.g. Toone, 1981), but these are outside the scope of this paper. A psychological account (Pond, 1957) is that the repeated intrusions into consciousness of bizarre and alien seizure related experiences and affects could have deleterious effects on the patient's mental health, and prepare the ground for a later psychotic development. There are some data supporting this hypothesis. For example, patients with complex auras manifest more psychopathology than those with simple auras (Standage & Fenton, 1975). Patients with auras consisting of illusions, hallucinations, and complex automatisms are at increased risk for psychosis relative to other types of auras (Jensen & Larsen 1979).

SOCIOECONOMIC STATUS

Being able to obtain and maintain a satisfactory job and an income is obviously relevant to an individual's psychosocial functioning, if only because unemployment introduces economic stresses, and may reduce the opportunities for social interaction, leisure activities and such. Unfortunately, unemployment and underemployment of people with epilepsy is much more frequent than in the general population. According to So and Penry (1981), the unemployment rate for people with epilepsy is two times the national average in the U.S. Many individuals with epilepsy experience problems finding work (Fraser, 1980, gives an estimate of 50%), and it is by no means uncommon that people loose their job because of seizures. It is no surprise that people with epilepsy generally have lower than average income.

The relationship between epilepsy and lower socioeconomic status is complex. The characteristics of the seizures may be such that they limit an individual's employment opportunities. Bothersome personality or behaviour characteristics may contribute to difficulties with employment. Cognitive functioning may be a significant factor in determining successful or unsuccessful employment status. Neuropsychological investigations of epilepsy have found, for example, that measures of higher cortical function predict vocational status and adequacy of psychosocial functioning (Dikmen & Morgan, 1980; Dodrill, 1980). Also, epilepsy continues to be associated with considerable stigma and ignorance, manifesting itself in various forms of social discrimination, e.g. difficulties in obtaining a driver's license, discrimination in obtaining employment (Fraser, 1980), difficulty in obtaining all types of insurance. The National Commission for the Control of Epilepsy and its Consequences (1978) has outlined the societal sanctions in greater detail. Such sanctions are conducive to social exclusion and ostracism, which may result in limited opportunities for extended social contact. Public attitudes towards epilepsy and misconceptions about this condition may go a long way in accounting for the difficulties experienced in getting employment.

Socioeconomic status is a potential confounding variable in studies on the psychological impact of epilepsy. For example, lower socioeconomic groups tend to manifest a higher rate of various psychiatric disturbances, including psychosis, relative to higher socioeconomic status groups. The reported rates of psychopathology may thus be seriously confounded by socioeconomic status effects, as much of the relevant literature is derived from individuals attending clinics which serve a high proportion of unemployed and other disadvantaged populations in the U.S. Increased scores on measures of psychopathology and/or measures of psychosocial complications that are obtained from samples selected at institutions serving groups with low socioeconomic status, may be more closely related to the effects of unemployment, poverty and such than to the effects of epilepsy per se (Hermann & Whitman, 1984). Variables reflecting socioeconomic status are thus extremely relevant to any index of psychosocial functioning in epilepsy.

CONCLUDING REMARKS

A very heterogeneous group psychosocial problems is associated with epilepsy. These include, among others, personality and behaviour difficulties, educational problems, changed affect, psychiatric problems, difficulties in finding work, frightening experiences during seizures, and popular misconceptions and prejudices still surrounding epilepsy. As we have noted in the foregoing, a number of standardized, reliable and well validated instruments are available "off the shelf" for providing assessment in some of these problem areas, e.g. various personality inventories and depression scales. Though these instruments were not developed with epilepsy in mind, there is no reason why they could not be applied in this context as well, perhaps after some minor modifications. However, the available instruments obviously do not cover the whole range of psychosocial problems in epilepsy. For example, parental attitudes and expectations, seizure related experiences or perceived stigma and discrimination because of the epilepsy all represent areas of concern that are highly specific to epilepsy. An adequate evaluation of such problems requires measures specifically designed for epilepsy.

REFERENCES

Aldenkamp, A.P. (1983). Epilepsy and learning behavior. In M. Parsonage, A.G. Craig, R.H.E. Grant and A.A. Ward (Eds.), Advances in epileptology: the XIVth Epilepsy International Symposium. New York: Raven Press.

Aldenkamp, A. P., Van Wieringen, A., Alpherts, W. C. J., Van Emde Boas, W., Haverkort, E., De Vries, J. & Meinardi, H. (1990). Double-blind placebo-controlled neuropsychological and neurophysiological investigations with oxiracetam (CGP 21690E) in memory impaired patients with epilepsy. Neuro-psychobiology, 14, 90–101.

Alpherts, W.C.J. & Aldenkamp, A.P. (1990). Computerized neuropsychological assessment of cognitive functioning in children with epilepsy. Epilepsia, 31(suppl 4), 35–40.

Bear, D. M. (1979). Temporal lobe epilepsy: A syndrome of sensory-limbic hyperconnection. Cortex, 15, 357–384.

Bear, D. M. & Fedio, P. (1977). Quantitative analysis of interictal behaviour in temporal lobe epilepsy. Archives of Neurology, 34, 454–467.

Dikmen, S. & Morgan, S. F. (1980). Neuropsychological factors related to employability and occupational status in persons with epilepsy. Journal of Nervous and Mental Disease, 168, 236–240.

Dodrill, C. B. (1980). Interrelationships between neuropsychological data and social problems in epilepsy. In R. Canger, F. Angeleri, & J. K. Penry (Eds.), Advances in epileptology: XIth epilepsy international symposium (pp. 191–197). New-York: Raven Press.

Fenton, G. W. (1981). Personality and behavioral disorders in adults with epilepsy. In E. H. Reynolds & M. R. Trimble (Eds.), Epilepsy and psychiatry (pp. 77–91). Edinburgh: Churchill Livingstone.

Fraser, R. T. (1980). Vocational aspects of epilepsy. In B. P. Hermann (Ed.), A multidisciplinary handbook of epilepsy (pp. 74–105). Springfield Ill: Charles C. Thomas.

Gibbs, F. A. & Stamps, F.W. (1953). Epilepsy handbook. Springfield Ill: Charles C. Thomas.

Hermann, B. F. (1979). psychopathology in epilepsy and learned helplessness. Medical Hypotheses, 5, 723–729.

Hermann, B. P., & Whitman. (1984). Behavioral and personality correlates of epilepsy: A review, methodological critique, and conceptual model. Psychological Bulletin, 95, 451–497.

Hermann, B. P., Dikmen, S., Schwarz, M. S. & Karnes, W. E. (1982). Psychopathology in TLE patients with ictal fear: A quantitative investigation. Neurology, 32, 7–11.

Jensen, I. & Larsen, J. K. (1979). Psychoses in drug resistant temporal lobe epilepsy. Journal of Neurology Neurosurgery and Psychiatry, 42, 948–954.

Lechtenberg, R. (1984). Epilepsy and the family. Boston: Harvard University Press.

Long, C. G. & Moore, J. L. (1979). Parental expectations for their epileptic children. Journal of Child Psychology and Psychiatry, 20, 299–312.

Mittan, R. J. & Locke, G. E. (1982). Fear of seizures: Epilepsy's forgotten problem. Urban Health, January/February, 40–41.

National Commission for the Control of Epilepsy and its Consequences (1978). Plan for the nationwide action on epilepsy (DHEW Publications No NIH 78–276), Washington DC.

Pond, D. A. (1975). Psychiatric aspects of epilepsy. Journal of the Indian Medical Profession, 3, 1441–1451.

Seidenberg, M., Beck, N., Geisser, M., Giordani, B., Sackellaris, J.C., Berent, S., Dreifuss, F.E., Boll, T.J. (1986). Academic achievement of children with epilepsy. Epilepsia, 29, 753–759.

Seligman, M. E. P. (1975). Helplessness. San Francisco: Freeman.

So, E. L. & Penry, J. K. (1981). Epilepsy in adults. Annals of Neurology, 9, 3–16.

Standage, K. F. & Fenton, G. W. (1975). Psychiatric symptom profiles of patients with epilepsy: A controlled investigation. Psychological medicine, 5, 152–160.

Strauss, E. (1989). Ictal and interictal manifestations of emotions in epilepsy. In F. Boller & J. Grafman (Eds.), Handbook of neuropsychology, Vol 3, (pp. 315–344). Amsterdam: Elsevier.

Thompson, P.J. (1987). Educational attainment in children and young people with epilepsy. In J. Oxley & G. Stores (Eds.), Epilepsy and Education (pp. 15–24). London: The Medical Tribune Group.

Toone, B. K. (1981). Psychoses of epilepsy. In E. H. Reynolds & M. R. Trimble (Eds.), Epilepsy and psychiatry (pp. 113–137). Edinburgh: Churchill Livingstone.

Treiman, D. M. (1986). Epilepsy and violence: medical and legal issues. Epilepsia, 27(Suppl. 2), 77–104.

Treiman, D. M. & Delgado-Escueta, A. V. (1983). Violence and epilepsy: A critical review. In T. A. Pedley & B. S. Meldrum (Eds.), Recent advances in epilepsy, Vol 1, (pp. 179–209). London: Churchill Livinstone.

Ward, F. & Bower, B. D. (1978). A study of certain social aspects of epilepsy in childhood. Developmental Medicine and Child Neurology, 39(Suppl), 1–50.

Waxman, S. G. & Geschwind, N. (1975). The interictal behavior syndrome of temporal lobe epilepsy. Archives of General Psychiatry, 32, 1580–1588.

West, P. (1979). An investigation into the social construction and consequences of the label epilepsy. Sociological Review, 27, 719–741.

Whitman, S., Hermann, B. P. & Gordon, A. (1984). Psychopathology in epilepsy: How great is the risk? Biological Psychiatry, 19, 213–236.

A CLINIMETRIC APPROACH FOR PSYCHOSOCIAL EFFECTS

Albert P. Aldenkamp, Ph.D.

Instituut voor Epilepsiebestrijding "Meer en Bosch"/"de Cruquiushoeve"
and Department for Paediatric Psychology
State University of Leyden
P.O. Box 21
2100 AA Heemstede
The Netherlands

INTRODUCTION

A clinimetric approach to the psychosocial consequences of epilepsy would assist us in finding an overall index for the evaluation of effects of the disease in long term follow-up studies. Thus, one of the advantages of such an index is that it would enable us to measure a patient repeatedly and to plot an individual 'illness career' over time (Feinstein, 1967; 1987).

Secondly, it would give us a measure that can easily be transferred to different situations, thereby increasing the possibility to compare groups of patients in different situations. Thus, the psychosocial effects of epilepsy could be compared with the psychosocial effects of other types of chronic illness.

In general, the reasons that have been mentioned to apply clinimetrics for designing clinical indexes (Cramer et al., 1983; Mattson et al., 1985; Baker et al., 1991; Wijsman et al., 1991) are also valid for an index of psychosocial effects. It allows to quantify data, it gives a comprehensive measurement that expresses complex and interconnected factors and it increases standardization and comparability.

The overall review of our current knowledge with regard to psychosocial assessment has been addressed by Vermeulen and Canger (1993; this volume).

This contribution to the discussion aims at finding rules that may help us to design clinimetric approaches for the psychosocial consequences of epilepsy.

Quantitative Assessment in Epilepsy Care, Edited by H. Meinardi et al.
Plenum Press, New York, 1993

CONSIDERATIONS FOR A CLINIMETRIC APPROACH TO PSYCHOSOCIAL EFFECTS

When discussing a clinimetric approach to psychosocial effects we refer to the outcome as a scale, an index, or a clinimetric measurement. In all cases we define this as an ordered registration of psychosocial functions that are quantified and may result in an overall endscore or several indices.

The label 'psychosocial' is used here to indicate both psychic and social reactions to the illness, covering a broad area of functions, such as mood, personality structure, school progress, coping behaviour or working habits.

State-Trait factors

The first consideration is that a clinimetric approach to psychosocial effects cannot be aimed at state and trait aspects simultaneously without specific adjustments in the index. Both aspects for example could be addressed in separate subscales. State aspects pertain to the direct 'ictal' psychosocial effects of the seizures such as headache, confusion, mood problems, experienced by the patients after, immediately before, or in direct relationship with the seizures. State aspects are difficult to measure as there nature is, by definition, transient.

Trait aspects are more easy to measure. They relate to more stable 'interictal' psychosocial aspects and are probably caused by the condition or by epilepsy-related factors such as drug treatment.

State and trait aspects are generally related, but constitute different areas of functioning.

Selection of Attributes

Next, the selection of proper attributes, to be included in the clinimetric psychosocial index comes into consideration. This aspect, of course, varies with the specific issue for which the index is used.

The clinimetric approach may be applicable to produce data that may assist in diagnostic procedures, for example with the differential diagnosis epilepsy versus pseudoepileptic seizures. The diagnosis pseudoepileptic seizures often requires the use of data about the personality structure, such as measures of self esteem and locus of control (Aldenkamp & Mulder, 1990). A psychosocial index may help us in summarising such a complex set of interconnecting factors.

Another application is to standardize the evaluation of patients' reactions to medical interventions, such as before and after functional epilepsy surgery or before and after the start of treatment with a new type of antiepileptic drug. In the first case, the index must certainly contain factors that refer to localized function impairment, such as speech disorders or memory impairment. If the index aims at evaluating side-effect of antiepileptic treatment then the scale must contain some global measures of cognitive function (especially 'speed factors') and possibly mood factors.

An important area in which the clinimetric approach will certainly be helpful, is the long-term follow-up of inpatients in long-stay treatment. This approach has been used by us to monitor behaviour in long-term clinical treatment of mentally handicapped patients with epilepsy. For some of these patients a special follow-up procedure may be necessary, especially as their behaviour does not require immediate attention. In such patients depressive reactions may remain unnoticed for a long period, unless careful monitoring is carried out. In our centre a clinimetric approach was used to evaluate success/failure rate of a rehabilitation unit for adolescents (Aldenkamp & Van Rossum, 1987). Such indexes aim at evaluating overall functioning and require subscales for social contacts, activity, personality make-up, signs of depression etc..

Finally, a clinimetric scale may serve as a tool in the decision making process in clinical practice ("can this patient comply with..."). In such a scale, certainly some aspects of daily life function must be included, such as school progress, working habits etc..

Our proposal is to use a scale for each specific occasion. This 'tailor-made strategy' may seem superficial, but it prevents that we try to use one scale for each separate issue, which undoubtedly raises problems of validity and clinical relevance (Aldenkamp et al., 1992; Crocker & Algina, 1986; Cronbach, 1989; Feldt & Brennan, 1990).

Form of the Psychosocial Index

Psychosocial indexes, following clinimetrical principles, can use a variety of forms:

- *Self-reports*, evaluating the opinion of the patient himself. Of course this type of assessment suffers from the pitfalls of using patient complaints in general. In general a large discrepancy is found between patient complaints about his psychosocial function and results of psychosocial assessment procedures (Aldenkamp et al., 1992). It would therefore be naive to rely exclusively on the opinion of the patients. Patients may be fully unaware of cognitive impairment, such as with transient amnesia, despite their clear failure during investigations. Some of the disadvantages can be overcome by using additional spouse or parent ratings. However there is no general rule how to handle discrepancies between patient and spouse complaints. Self-reports can take any given form such as visual analogue scales, questionnaires, monitoring lists, diaries etc..

- *Checklists* are mostly physician based instruments and aim at increasing the standardization and reliability of the clinical judgment. The checklists can be administered by the neurologist, the psychologist or a research assistant and can be complemented with (semi)structured interviews.

- *Investigations or assessment procedures*, using objective parameters to measure certain dimensions or factors. Such procedures can result in one index or in separate indices for each specific area such as cognitive function, behaviour, social functioning and personality (including psychiatric symptoms). Mostly these type of scales measure domains of functions that can be observed by the clinician.

Validity

The question of the validity of such indexes is still open. This is a serious obstacle for the development of a clinimetric procedure for psychosocial effects as it must compete with several instruments used in standard clinical practice, such as depression lists, anxiety scales, personality inventories, some of them with excellent psychometric qualities.

Probably the best procedure is to combine these procedures until the validity of the clinimetric index against these standard procedures has been confirmed (this procedure is called criterion-related validation). It then has to be questioned whether the psychosocial index can be used in all situations in which the clinicians have to judge the psychosocial consequences of the seizures or of the epilepsy.

A problem connected with the validity testing is that most clinimetric procedures are discontinuous scales, i.e. use a kind of 'cut-off' score: scores above a certain level are considered a sign for dysfunctioning. Most standard tests for psychosocial functioning are constructed as (semi)continuous scales, which give a ranking of functioning. The comparison of results obtained with such different methods will be rather difficult.

For a review of the statistical procedures related to the validity of such scales see Crocker & Algina (1986), Cronbach (1989), Feldt & Brennan (1990).

A Psychosocial Index 'Stand Alone' or Included in the Clinical Index

The next option that needs a decision is whether psychosocial factors have to be included in a general clinical index or must be constructed as a 'stand alone scale'. An example of the first option is the Veterans Administration Clinimetrical Procedure by Cramer and colleagues (Cramer et al., 1983; Mattson et al., 1985). In this index the physician assesses affect, mood and cognitive function with two questions. However a supplementary neuropsychological battery is administered to the patients. Between the neuropsychological battery, 'The Behavioral Toxicity Battery', and the outcomes of the questions a high correlation was found (Mattson, personal communication). Nevertheless it may be questioned whether such a limited number of questions can really cover the broad domain of psychosocial functions that are important in patients with chronic epilepsy.

An excellent example of a 'stand alone' procedure is the Washington Psychosocial Seizure Inventory (WPSI) by Dodrill (1980). The WPSI is a 132-item questionnaire requiring yes/no answers. It is specifically designed to evaluate psychosocial problems of patients with epilepsy over 16 years of age. The WPSI gives a total index score for the impact of epilepsy on psychosocial functioning ('Overall psychosocial functioning') and allows for subscale analysis (a profile is obtained for seven dimensions, such as emotional adjustment, financial status and vocational adjustment).

Both procedures have their benefits. The main benefit of the overall procedure is, that it gives one comprehensive index that takes into account all kind of clinical information, the psychosocial status included. The cost is the loss of information, that may be dramatic when a differential diagnosis is needed. The benefit of a scale with several indices for subscales is that it allows for profile analysis that may allow a more sophisticated judgement of several domains of functioning simultaneously. However it creates the problem of coupling two different sets of information. This is especially important when the scale has to be used in drug trials.

THE DEVELOPMENT OF A PSYCHOSOCIAL INDEX

All successful scales have been developed from an existing starting point. This procedures allows to use a 'gold standard' for the development of the new scale. The best rationale would therefore be to start with an existing scale that should be tailored to the specific needs of the clinician or the trial in which the scale has to be used. Currently there are three types of indexes or scales that can be used as a good starting point.

- The first starting point is the VA-scale (Cramer et al., 1983; Mattson et al., 1985). We may use this scale, although this requires that more items concerning affect and cognition should be included in the scale.
- The second option is to use the WPSI, that has the advantage of being cross-cultural validated (Dodrill, 1980). Moreover is has proven to be sensitive for at least the use in the follow-up after neurosurgery and general assessment of patients with chronic epilepsy.
- The third option is to use general indicators. Deyo (1984) and Jette (1980) classify the measures giving indexes for psychosocial effects of chronic disease into four categories:

  a) Disease-specific instruments for evaluating the impact of the specific illness on psychosocial functioning (most scales have been developed for cancer or arthritis).

  b) Instruments based on the 'quality of care' concept such as the 'Problem Status scale'. Such scales evaluate the judgments about the treatment.

  c) Scales that focus on daily life function, such as "The Index of Activities for Daily Living" (Jette, 1980).

  d) General Health Status Measures. Deyo (1984) concludes that only for instruments, classified in this last category, validity studies have been carried out.

A promising option within this last category and used in a pilot study on patients with epilepsy by our group is the Sickness Impact Profile (Bergner et al., 1981; Bergner 1988; Gilson et al., 1975; Pollard et al., 1976), that gives a general index of sickness impairment as subjectively assessed by the patients. Other examples are the General Health Questionnaire and the Nottingham Health Profile.

These kinds of measures can also be classified in the group of 'quality of life measures'. Quality of life is ".... a multidimensional construct which covers physical, emotional, mental, social and behavioral components of well-being and function as perceived by patients and observers" (Anderson, 1992). A vital concept in the 'quality of life' approach "is that health is not merely the absence of disease, nor merely survival, nor even disease control alone, but the active promotion of well-being" "....it serves to transcend the mainstream medical model approach and to distinguish the predicament of biology from the experience of illness" (Anderson, 1992). Although a number of trials have been carried out, using experimental 'quality of life scales', as yet, no sufficient validated 'quality of life scale' is available for epilepsy or any other chronic illness.

CONCLUSION

It seems extremely difficult to include parameters of psychosocial functioning into a clinimetric index: First 'trait' aspects must be distinguished from 'state' aspects. Secondly, it is probably not possible to find a limited number of key items that cover all domains of psychosocial functioning (or are representative for the full domain of psychosocial functioning) and are also applicable in all issues. Consequently, this would lead to a large number of psychosocial indices that all will have to meet the key criteria of psychometrics: validity and reliability.

The clinimetric approach therefore is best encouraged:

- by selecting one issue to develop an index, such as the detection of side-effects of antiepileptic drugs. This instrument may then be used experimentally in research. We would benefit from the psychometric procedure applied to such a scale, as it would consequently serve as the 'gold standard' to develop new instruments.

- by using a physician-based instrument, in stead of asking a patient to evaluate his/her own psychosocial functioning. The use of patient-based instruments adds new problems (such as discrepancies between patient reports and results of assessment procedures) in this already rather complex area.

- by combining the index with normal assessment procedures, such as cognitive tests, personality tests, mood rating scales etc.. Only if the index has shown its value against these measures (used as 'gold standards') a clinimetric approach may be uncoupled from standard testing procedures.

- by starting with an existing 'stand alone' instrument. Although a vast body of research on 'quality of life measures' is carried out and undoubtedly holds a promise, we strongly advise to start the clinimetric approach with the only existing instrument for psychosocial follow-up of patients with epilepsy, the WPSI.

REFERENCES

Aldenkamp, A.P. & van Rossum, A.W. Effects of Pedagogic Strategies in the treatment of children with Epilepsy. In: P. Wolf, M. Dam, D. Janz & F.E. Dreifuss (eds). Advances in Epileptology, 1987, pp. 621–627. Raven Press, New York.

Aldenkamp, A.P. & Mulder, O.G. Some considerations on diagnosis and treatment of pseudo-epileptic seizures in adolescents. Intern. Journ. of Adolescent Medicine and Health, 1990, 4(2), 81–91

Aldenkamp AP, Vermeulen J, Alpherts WCJ et al. Validity of computerized testing: patient dysfunction and complaints versus measured changes. In: W.E. Dodson & M. Kinsbourne, Assessment of cognitive function in epilepsy, 1992, pp. 51–68. Demos, New York.

Anderson, L. 'Quality of Life'. Epilepsy International News, 1992.

Baker GA, Smith DF, Dewey M et al. The development of a seizure severity scale as an outcome measure in epilepsy. Epilepsy Research, 1991, 8, 245–251.

Bergner M, Bobbitt RA, Carter WB & Gilson B. The Sickness Impact Profile: development and final revision of a Health Status Measure. Medical care, 1981, 19, 787.

Bergner M. Development, testing and use of the Sickness Impact Profile. In: Walker SR & Rosser MR (eds) Quality of Life: Assessment and Application. MTP Press Limited, 1988.

Cramer JA, Mattson RH, Smith DB et al. A method of quantification for the evaluation of antiepileptic drug therapy. Neurology, 1983, 33, 26–37.

Crocker L & Algina J. Introduction to classical and modern test theory. Holt, Rinehart and Winston, New York, 1986.

Cronbach LJ. Essentials of Psychological Testing, Harper, 1989, New York.

Deyo RA. Measuring functional outcomes in therapeutic trials for chronic disease. Controlled clinical trials, 1984, 5, 223–240.

Dodrill CB. An objective method for the assessment of psychological and social problems among epileptics. Epilepsia, 1980, 21, 123–135.

Feinstein AR. Indexes and criteria for the therapeutic response. In: Clinical Judgement, Huntingon, pp. 247–263. Kreiger Publishing, New York, 1967.

Feinstein AR. Clinimetrics. Yale University Press, New Haven, 1987.

Feldt LS & Brennan RL. Reliability. In: Linn RL (ed.) Educational Measurement. New York, 1990.

Gilson BS, Gilson JS & Bergner M. The Sickness Impact Profile. Development of an outcome measure of health care. Am. Journ. Pub. Health, 1975, 65, 1304–1310.

Jette AM. Health Status Indicators: Their utility in chronic disease evaluation research. Journ Chron. Disease, 1980, 33, 567–579.

Mattson RH, Cramer JA, Collins JF. et al. Comparison of Carbamazepine, Phenobarbitone, Phenytoin and Primidone in partial and secondarily generalized tonic clonic seizures. New Engl. Journ of Med., 1985, 313, 145–151.

Pollard WE, Bobbitt RA & Bergner M. The Sickness Impact Profile: Reliability of a health status measure. Med. Care, 1976, 14, 146–155.

Vermeulen J and Canger R. Psychosocial Consequences of Epilepsy. This Volume.

Wijsman DJP, Hekster YA, Keyser A, et al. Clinimetrics and epilepsy care. Pharmaceutisch Weekblad; Scientific Edition, 1991, 13, 182–188.

GENERAL DISCUSSION OF THE PART PLAYED BY HEALTH STATUS, ADVERSE EFFECTS OF TREATMENT AND PSYCHOSOCIAL FACTORS IN THE CONSTRUCTION OF INDEXES

RENIER: I have not heard a definition of what health is, we are speaking about health status, but what is health? Did we use the definition that health is a lack of disease or a lack of signs and symptoms, or is health a state of physical, social and mental well-being? If we are speaking about well-being, this is a much more subjective impression of people and needs a patient-based scale. We know the type of patient who reacts to seizure suppression by saying "the treatment robbed me of my epilepsy." For him it was not a good result that he had no seizures as his pattern of life had completely depended on his seizures and now life felt empty. Another remark I have to make is: we discussed seizure frequency, and then severity of seizures, now we add a third component, health status. The topic becomes more and more complicated. In fact in most clinical trials of anti-epileptic drugs we do not admit patients with other diseases or pregnant women. If indexes are only to be used in research it seems there would be no place to discuss the health aspect.

CRAMER: The modifying factor of an illness in our scale is not the issue of a chronic concomitant illness, but rather an occasional viral illness that occurred. The weighting accounted for the fact that for some individuals the fever would affect their seizure frequency. As far as the dissecting out what is the impact of epilepsy or a concomitant chronic illness on the quality of life of the patient, I fear that that is an impossible task.

MEINARDI: It has been mentioned that depression, which is frequently associated with epilepsy, might influence the outcome of the seizure severity scale.

DUNCAN: By our scale it should not affect it at all. The scales, the individual scores, are based upon objective data i.e. the answer to the question "how long does it take you to return to normal after a seizure?." There is no component in our seizure severity scale of perception of "how do you feel," so feeling depressed should not make any difference.

MEINARDI: The issue raised is that items measured by the scale like "how long does it take you to return to normal after a seizure?" might be affected by a concomitant depression.

Quantitative Assessment in Epilepsy Care, Edited by H. Meinardi et al.
Plenum Press, New York, 1993

163

BAKER: You are right, it is an important issue, we actually looked at how depression may interact with patients' perception of their seizure, using our seizure severity scale and using a well validated scale of depression, however it was not a significant predictor of the outcome, it did not account for a significant amount of the variance.

CRAMER: We used an entirely separate, neuropsychological test battery—the Profile Of Mood Scale—in addition to our seizure severity rating scales and our adverse effect rating scales. I do not think it is pertinent to the specific seizure severity scales that we have talked about, it is another issue, because you do not know if the patient's clinical status, including whether his depression is changing and that is really the issue.

ALDENKAMP: Dr Baker we know that patients who are depressed, complain more about their somatic problems. On pain scores it appears as if they feel more pain, yet they do not experience more severity of their seizures according to your severity scale. How do you explain that? Is it a problem of the sensitivity of your scale?

BAKER: The scale we used was the Snave Hospital Anxiety and Depression Scale, and of the population that we looked at, 15% actually fell into the level of clinical depression. That is probably equitable to most previous studies that looked at depression in patients with chronic epilepsy. So that scale was sensitive enough to be accounting for the variance in the seizure severity scale if depression did influence outcome. However, it does not appear to substantially account for the variance between individuals on the seizure severity scale.

CRAMER: We have to consider that we are often looking at change within an individual over time. So even if a patient has some chronic pain problem, if we assume a level of constancy of this without known exacerbations, and we look at an epilepsy scale longitudinally over time, every six months or every year, with or without an intervention, we should be able to attribute the change to the epilepsy and we can close our eyes to the other disease.

MEINARDI: Dr Duncan the title of your presentation was the clinimetric approach to individualization of treatment. I gather that you are not so much in favour of this, because you feel that a scale might even more confuse the issue of tailor made treatment because the scales are often designed to compare groups and not to assess individuals. However, would you not agree that it might be useful to have a scale which is automatically recorded at each consultation and which has a danger marker level. The same as the red light on your dashboard that starts to blink every time something is wrong with your cooling system.

DUNCAN: I think it is important to separate research issues from questions of routine clinical management. We agree it is important to measure seizure numbers and seizure severity in both situations. I do not think that the efficacy of anti-epileptic drug treatment in an individual will be usefully measured with a single composite score. To pursue the motor car analogy, there are separate warning lights for temperature, oil, fuel and brakes and this is much more useful than a single warning light that indicates that there is some problem, but you do not know what it is.

MEINARDI: A point raised again and again is lack of golden standards. It was suggested that like in a cross-over trial one should compare two periods one before the use of a scale and one during which the scale is used. If no improvement in current clinical practice can be demonstrated after the introduction of the scale there is no use for it, is there? For example is the Chalfont scale improving clinical management?

SPILKER: I would like to clarify the comments on golden standards. It seems that here the term is being used differently from what most people do. You were using the term golden standard in terms of usefulness: "It will be a useful measure, improve clinical practise," but that has nothing to do with the definition of the term "golden standard." A golden standard means something that is universally agreed as being a definitive term of diagnosis such as used for autopsy material, biopsy material or a laboratory test that provides information universally agreed upon; or it might be another test like the Hamilton Scale for Depression about which there is consensus that it measures what it intends to.

DUNCAN: Anyway I think I'm not in a position to answer the question whether or not the Chalfont scale will assist clinical management. We are still in the assessment phase of reproducibility, consistency and validity. Once we have full validation we can start to employ the results.

MEINARDI: The question under debate is whether the scales presented should serve to improve clinical management or are they only applicable as a research instrument?

MATTSON: We developed our scales as a research tool and we have used it as such. Nevertheless, it reflects actual clinical practice correlating with the point when the physician deemed it appropriate to alter medication because he was not satisfied with the ongoing therapy.

MEINARDI: To assess the future impact of clinimetric methods on quality of clinical care will not be easy. Remember that Rodin showed in his book on prognosis in 1968 that up till then not more than 40% of people treated for epilepsy would attain remission. Recent papers quote percentages of up to 70%. Some papers have been ascribing this improvement in prognosis of the past twenty years to the introduction of therapeutic drug monitoring in epileptology. Yet some people are critical about measuring serum levels, insisting they really do not improve clinical practise as physicians would tend to treat sub-therapeutic or toxic **levels** instead of seizures. When we are constructing clinimetric scales the same may happen. In fact the serum level of an anti-epileptic drug is a kind of scale. It may not be easy to prove whether the clinimetric scale has a positive or negative impact.

CHADWICK: Surely these scales have little use in routine clinical practice. I would have great reservations about the need for a "red light" in a doctor-patient relationship. If there is a need for that kind of red light, you got a bad doctor sitting on the other side of the table.

MATTSON: It was said earlier that in view of the increasing concern with quality of care an instrument like this one might be very helpful to measure just that.

CHADWICK: In that circumstance, you are asking a specific research question about the provision of care. You are not using it to modulate your routine clinical practise, within an individual doctor-patient relationship.

MEINARDI: A question raised was to find out to what extend laboratory data should be part of our clinimetric scales. Or if put the other way around the question was: "How much assistance is provided by the laboratory in judging the effects of drug treatment. In particular do clinicians manage the possible problems with adverse effects resulting from the drug treatment by taking account of laboratory data." In fact Dr Mattson has pointed out several times that the clinimetric index is more a kind of final accounting of what has happened, all the decisions were made independently therefore perhaps these laboratory data that are meant to assist the clinician are not needed in an index.

MATTSON: The index, or better still the rating forms that have to be filled out provide relatively uniform information from different places. Also if you want to know if one drug is better than another, then the only way you can actually have scientifically valid numbers, is to record them. If we asked "How are you," by using this scale it helped to give us the impression that the people on carbamazepine were a little better off than the people on valproate. So it didn't drive our decisions, but it did help give us information that may assist other people in drug selection.

ALDENKAMP: To proceed with our discussion about golden, silver or bronze standards, did you look at the correlation between your toxicity score and the behavioral toxicity battery, which was supplementary administered to the patient. Was there some correlation between those two measurements?

MATTSON: Yes there was a correlation. Dennis Smith has looked at this, in some detail, and there was also some correlation between the findings in the behavioral test battery and the reports of the clinician and the patient as to, say mood or cognitive disturbances. They were a little more borderline at least they did not reach significance levels. In terms of validation, I think it is a very important that the design of this rating scale came from literally a dozen epileptologists who worked with it over a period maybe of about a year and had it refined and refined,so people were in good agreement that it was workable and corresponded to what we as clinicians thought was appropriate. Then it was pilot tested in the type of study for which it was designed. After some four thousand patient visits, we did an interim analysis of the use of the rating scales, to see if the score of fifty, that we considered to correspond with an unacceptable outcome, correlated with when people were taken off drug, and in fact it did.

MEINARDI: How well did the laboratory data on the serum levels of AED correlate with your toxicity data?

MATTSON: Not too well. In general, as you know, the problem with this I think is explained, that some people with epilepsy, even without treatment don't have seizures, some people with *optimal* AED therapy continue to have seizures, and so, trying to correlate the levels and the outcome is always pretty difficult.

CRAMER: In an analysis I presented at the American Epilepsy Society Meeting this year, I showed that there was very little corroboration of a so called therapeutical target range with these data but the reason is largely because we didn't make our patients sick enough. In a research mode this would have been a nice opportunity to push the dose to make people really sick so we could test the hypothesis, but we didn't. The whole emphasis was to maintain patients as is usual in clinical practice, so we stopped short when they reached a modicum of toxicity for that individual. Whether it was the red light going on on the dashboard because of a clinical feeling or the scale score, the physician responded by lowering the dose. That thwarted the opportunity to really do a good evaluation of the drug levels versus the toxicity. Another issue as part of the study is that the physicians did not see the exact drug level because it was a blinded study. What we did instead, for each drug we devised a range, and sub divided it into "low, mid, and high," so that the phenytoin level of 10–20 micrograms per ml, was divided into a low of 10–12, mid of 13–16, and a high of 17–20. All the physician was told was e.g., "The drug you use is in the high range."

MEINARDI: A question was raised about the impact that the knowledge of the blood level had on the clinical decision making in the VA study.

MATTSON: This kind of information was mainly useful in the start up phase. Trying to get them into what we feel was a reasonable dose to give a fair test to the drug. After people were on the drug, that information was rarely of any use. As I indicated, the decision as to whether to increase dose was determined by the occurrence of persisting seizures or to reduce if people were having unacceptable adverse effects.

KASTELEIJN: Could this be due to the type of information provided by the laboratory e.g., only trough levels. Would it not be better to use the trough and the peak levels together, and correlate the difference between the two with seizure counts and toxicity scales?

MATTSON: I don't think there's any doubt that the ability to do dose response, kind of studies, to look at peaks, troughs, and look at this in closer detail, would provide a lot more information, but that's as I must confess, a more elegant kind of study than we were able to carry out on some thousand people, and twelve different centres.

MEINARDI: Dr. Chadwick could you comment on the existence of covert adverse effects? Was there any information from your withdrawal studies about the presence or absence of this phenomenon.

CHADWICK: Yes, we got rather nice data from the Medical Research Council study. People in that study reported a very low incidence of side effects related to their drug treatment while they were taking drugs, because, of course, 80% of these people were on monotherapy, taking low doses of drug with low blood levels, because they have a very mild epilepsy. Continuing to take drugs made people worry a lot more about having epilepsy and gave them distress in a number of different psychosocial areas. So part of people's agenda very much is, as far as epilepsy is concerned, not only no seizures, but no drugs; epilepsy has not gone until both have gone. That is an important issue.

KEYSER: Aldenkamp in his contribution, made some remarks about placebo effects induced by doing clinimetric assessment in patients. I should like to come back to this because these remarks got lost, at least nobody made a comment.

ALDENKAMP: My point was that when it comes to evaluating psychosocial behaviour through a clinimetric approach, the approach should be very short, otherwise it gives more attention to the patient than a regular visit to another department not using clinimetrics. So the patient tends to feel more comfortable, he gets more attention and it has been proved, once and again, that the fact that the patients are asked about their behaviour or psychosocial problems that worry them, also influences their reactions, and their perception how life is going on. It is actually a danger of each type of assessment of patients whether you use personality tests or whatever, but in these kind of tests this problem is tackled by using a procedure with cross checking or other techniques. That has not been done yet in the clinimetric procedures which have been discussed. That what I meant.

SPILKER: If I understand what you said, you are worried about the effect of the patient–doctor interaction when clinimetric scales are introduced into the patient doctor communication. However, I would like to suggest that the physicians have a great variability because they ask the questions in term of evaluating patients already quite different from each other. Some of them are interviewing their patients in a much more aggressive way, others much more mildly. There's a lot of variation between physicians, whether or not extra attention is being paid to clinimetrics probably will not change this variation very much.

ALDENKAMP: Your point is well taken. I meant however, that it might be a problem in the testing phase of such a scale. When you use another measure to check your results, especially when you don't have a golden standard the assessment by your scale may be too mild just because of this placebo effect. Dr Cramer, did you discuss the scores with the patients and do you have any idea of the reaction of the patients once they found out about their level of functioning expressed in a number. And how was the behaviour of the physicians altered once the symptoms were graded?

CRAMER: We do not use these scores in patient-care or to advise patients what were their scores. Of course if you would tell the patient then you would have to teach them how to handle this information otherwise you might find what you sometimes observe when you tell a patient "it seems you have a slight (5 points) tremor," and immediately the tremor increases to a 20 point intensity. Dr Duncan do you plan to discuss your scores with the patients?

DUNCAN: We may say "On your major attacks you gave a score of 80 and your minor attacks you gave a score of 10. Could you tell me some more about the two types of seizures?"

REINIER: So you did use scales in communication as a physician?

DUNCAN: On the whole I favour a policy of "Glasnost." Yes we would intend to discuss the results.

JOHNSON: Can I just question something you said about the order in which you present the information to the patient. You report their scores, then you ask them to apply a relative severity measure to their seizure types; or you do it the other way round?

DUNCAN: In the validation exercise of the physician's scores, after writing the scores down but before comparing them, we ask the patients for their perception of the relative severity of their various types of seizures.

CRAMER: Dr Chadwick, you made a statement that there is a difference between efficacy and effectiveness. I think in a well planned clinical trial, efficacy and effectiveness should be identical.

CHADWICK: Yes, I accept what you say. The only reservation I have is, in view of the sample sizes needed. We limit our studies to a selected population to obtain the answer we want to know in the first place. The point that I was trying to make was that efficacy, means that this drug is better than the placebo in controlling seizures. That's the answer, looked for by industry and registration bodies. That doesn't matter to me at all. I want to know how this drug performs in routine clinical practise with all its clinical uncertainties and complicating factors. To measure that, I am using a scale measuring effectiveness.

MEINARDI: One way of putting it is that efficacy is simply assessing the statistical difference between treatment and placebo while effectiveness is the subjective evaluation of patient and physician that the treatment works. Often with respect to moving from efficacy to effectiveness of treatment, compliance is at stake (i.e., changing an efficacious treatment in an ineffective one). Another way of putting it is that efficacy addresses more the outcome of treatment on the disease and effectiveness the restitution of the patient to a life as if the disease had not been there. Dr Chadwick, do you include in your effectiveness scale also the price of the drug?

CHADWICK: I did not get into the whole issue of health economics because we are light years away from that, because in order to make some health economic assessment you first of all have to address the effect of the treatment might have on the global assessment and how much that costs to society and we are several steps away from that. I am not sure if anyone has an adequate conception to take those steps right now.

MEINARDI: I was speaking about affordability, because, nowadays in many countries—and perhaps soon in England too—patients have to pay for their drugs and that might be an element of effectiveness.

CHADWICK: Of course, it is something we all address in every health care system. Maybe a new drug might offer some benefits particularly in terms of less toxicity than the old ones. But it is a very difficult issue to address, whether all those small improvements in tolerability of the new drug justify the great expenses.

SPILKER: It seems when we look to phase I and II clinical trials these are along the line as Dr Chadwick described looking at efficacy. When we get to phase III I would suggest we are moving closer to measuring effectiveness. In phase III you really should be looking at clinical significance or clinical importance. When you develop your objectives for phase III trials that are looking at efficacy, there should also be concern with the question—how much of a change will be clinical important and not just how must of a change will be able to give us a P value of .05.

GLOBAL ASSESSMENTS IN EPILEPSY

David Chadwick, M.A., D.M., F.R.C.P.[1] and Ann Jacoby, B.A.[2]

[1]Professor of Neurology
Department of Neuroscience
Walton Centre for Neurology and Neurosurgery
Walton Hospital
Rice Lane, Liverpool L9 1AE

[2]Senior Research Assistant
Centre for Health Services Research
University of Newcastle Upon Tyne
21 Claremont Place, Newcastle Upon Tyne NE2 4AA
United Kingdom

INTRODUCTION

There can be no doubt that global assessments of outcome in epilepsy are necessary and that little work currently exists which is of relevance to the subject. The types of measure to be used will very much be determined by the questions being asked, as well as by whom the questions are being asked. Three main areas require examination.

(1) Assessments of new antiepileptic drugs often undertaken by the pharmaceutical industry for regulatory agencies.

(2) Clinically relevant pragmatic assessments of management policies (assessments of effectiveness rather than efficacy) usually addressing questions raised by the clinical community.

(3) Assessments of services and their cost-benefits often asked by purchasers and providers of services.

The purpose of this paper is to review the fundamental questions and existing progress in these areas. It will largely concentrate on more pragmatic assessments.

Quantitative Assessment in Epilepsy Care, Edited by H. Meinardi et al.
Plenum Press, New York, 1993

New Antiepileptic Drugs

The pharmaceutical industry is required to produce proof of efficacy in randomized placebo-controlled trial designs in order to obtain a licence for a new antiepileptic drug. Trials in this area are usually undertaken in highly selected populations of people with epilepsy who have frequent seizures in spite of existing antiepileptic drug treatment. Drugs are used for a short period in circumstances that diverge considerably from usual clinical practice. Tests of efficacy are largely based on tests of statistical significance rather than tests of clinically important changes. From the point of view of efficiency and power in these trials, the most sensitive measure will be detecting a change in the median (or mean) group change in seizure frequency (Van Belle & Temkin, 1981). Relatively small changes in a proportion of the patients studied may be sufficient to provide statistical evidence that an antiepileptic effect exists, but such an effect may not have great clinical relevance to the patients in the study.

New drug applications will also examine the adverse effects and complications of treatment with the new agent. Regulatory agencies and the pharmaceutical industry will have particular concerns about drugs which have potentially serious adverse effects or relatively narrow therapeutic windows. Regulatory agencies act on behalf of society as a whole to make global judgements as to whether the potential benefits of a new treatment outweigh the toxicity associated with the drug. Where a drug is introduced for treatment of a commonly fatal or poorly treated condition, a considerable degree of toxicity may be acceptable. In chronic conditions for which satisfactory treatment is already available, significant toxicity may prevent licensing.

Thus, in this setting an agency makes global judgements about a series of scientific experiments whose conclusions are subjected to statistical tests and assesses their views of the improved outcome against available information on the drug's toxicity. This kind of assessment, however, answers very few clinical questions. Once a drug is licensed clinicians will want to know how the relative efficacy and toxicity and global outcomes of the new agent compares with that of existing standard treatments.

Assessment of Management Policies

Patient-doctor contacts which involve treatment rather than diagnosis, are concerned with assessing the relative benefits and adverse effects of particular treatments. In routine clinical practice these issues are often dealt with in a very simple manner. The question "How are you?" to a patient attending a follow-up clinic because of epilepsy immediately invites him or her to make judgements firstly about the adequacy of control of the seizure disorder and secondly about any costs that may arise from the use of a particular treatment (which will usually be a pharmacological agent). Since routine clinical practice remains heavily dependent upon patients' perceptions of these issues it is important that the patient feels able to communicate his or her views and concerns to the clinician and that he or she feels adequately advised and informed about the potential benefits and risks of future changes in treatment. There can be little doubt that one of the major areas of patient dissatisfaction with doctor-patient contacts arise from failures in this two-way process.

In epilepsy, the emphasis over recent years has been to develop satisfactory measures of seizure "control." Most studies contain some measure of seizure frequency relevant to the population being studied. The measure to be used must, however, be relevant to patients. Perhaps the most useful and relevant measure in this area is the attainment of a clinically important remission of seizures for a two, three or five year period. This is likely to be the major goal of almost all patients presenting with epilepsy for the first time, particularly for those who have no other physical or mental handicap. In the MRC Antiepileptic Drug Withdrawal Study seizure recurrence clearly increased reported distress in the relevant domains of the Nottingham Health Profile, the amount people worried about their epilepsy and its effects on their everyday lives (Jacoby, 1992). However, for people with a long history of epilepsy who have never attained remission of their seizures, other measures of control may be important. A reduction of seizure frequency may be of value, though there is no evidence that the commonly used end-point of a 50% reduction in seizures with a new treatment is perceived as being important by people in this group (Smith et al, 1992). A reduction in the severity of seizures may be a useful alternative goal and satisfactory measures of seizure severity could enhance the sensitivities of clinical trials (Baker et al, 1991). We would argue that such measures should be patient-based because there is evidence that there may be discrepancies in assessment between professionals and patients (Slevin et al, 1988) as well as discrepancies between patients with the same disease state (Ziller, 1974). There is evidence from a population of people with intractable epilepsy that scales measuring psychological distress are more highly correlated with patient-based measures of seizure severity than with assessments of seizure frequency (Smith et al, 1991). Thus, research suggests that reliance on measures of control which are not based on patients' perceptions may lack clinical relevance.

Methods for ascertaining and quantifying adverse effects of treatments should also take account of patients' perceptions, yet in most clinical trials there are no standardised procedures used to elicit symptoms of adverse events. A scoring system has been developed by the VA study group (Cramer et al, 1983) and added to a seizure activity score to give a global score but this is an observer-based system that does not quantify the patients perceptions or the importance of symptoms or signs to that individual's life. The weighting involved in the system does not appear well validated.

There is, of course, a large literature on the potential effects of antiepileptic drugs on cognitive function, memory and behaviour but it is difficult to be certain whether small statistically significant changes in scales examining cognitive function and memory have any direct clinical relevance. Here again is a problem of a statistically significant change being of questionable clinical importance. Recent evidence suggests that monotherapy, (in groups of patients with mild drug-responsive epilepsy) with doses of standard antiepileptic drugs commonly used and highly effective, has few effects on a battery of psychometric scales (Meador et al, 1991). In the MRC Antiepileptic Drug Withdrawal Study, whilst only a small proportion of patients said that they had side-effects from antiepileptic drugs that they were taking, it was clear that there were a number of adverse psychosocial consequences of continuing to take antiepileptic drugs. There was, in fact, as much distress about continuing to take drugs as there was in having seizures during the course of follow-up and indeed a high proportion of patients who had seizures on withdrawal of treatment in the study had no regrets about attempting to come off antiepileptic drugs (Jacoby, Johnson, Chadwick, 1992). It seems clear that continuing to take antiepileptic drugs represents part of the process of stigmatisation associated with the diagnostic label of epilepsy (Scambler, 1989) and that many people do not feel that the label can be removed until the ultimate ideal is attained, that is—no fits and no drugs. It may be that clinicians have in the past made relatively naive assumptions about the patient's viewpoint in this area, and that conventional assessments miss this.

While it is clear, therefore, that global assessments must examine the issues of both control and adverse effects of treatment, it must be self-evident that the only person capable of making such judgements about the relative costs and benefits is the patient. It seems essential, therefore, that clinical trials should elicit their views. Unfortunately, though there is increasing emphasis in the literature on the need to do so (Cartwright, 1983; Drummond, 1987), relatively little work has been done in this area so far, particularly in epilepsy (Baker, PhD Thesis)

One measure which addresses both efficacy and adverse effects has been used by the VA study group (Mattson et al, 1985). They used retention-time in randomized groups, that is the proportion of patients randomized to a particular drug who remain on the drug with the passage of time. Such a measure reflects both efficacy and toxicity as does time to remission (6 months, 1 or 2 years) as long as withdrawals from randomization policies are treatment viewed as not attaining such a remission (Turnbull et al, 1985). Where such measures are used they will reflect patient perceptions as long as the trial concerned is pragmatic, reflecting clinical practice, so that the decision to withdraw a treatment reflects patients preferences rather than artificially imposed judgements peculiar to a clinical trial.

In clinical trials patients are often asked whether they consider themselves to have improved during the period of treatment. This kind of simple approach has some merit though no-one has examined correlations between patients perceptions of improvement and information about seizure-control and adverse effects during the treatment period. There is also evidence that relatively simple questions to patients can elicit meaningful answers. Thus, in the Antiepileptic Drug Withdrawal Study asking patients to rate how much they worried about their epilepsy was significantly related to their scores on scales measuring well-being, stigmatization, mastery, and self-esteem, and the patients who worried a lot about their epilepsy were also more likely to have had recent seizures or be taking antiepileptic drugs at the time of the questionnaire.

Thus, where more sophisticated methods of quality of life assessment are impractical, it may be sufficient to ask patients a small number of relatively simple questions which have been shown to correlate with other more complete measures. For example, a question which addresses patients' adjustment to their epilepsy in relation to a number of different aspects of their everyday life has been shown to correlate well with a number of previously validated psychological measures (Baker and Jacoby, in prep.). Indeed, simple answers to overall questions may be necessary to complement and allow interpretation of more sophisticated quality of life profiles.

Assessment of Service Provisions

Research in the field of epilepsy has tended to focus on the efficacy and side-effects of individual drugs and, to a lesser extent, on particular treatment policies. Only rarely, to our knowledge, has attention been paid to the way systems of care for people with epilepsy are provided, or to the views of the recipients of that care. This may be, in part, because the consumers of health care, dependent as they are upon the judgements and actions of professional staff, are relatively powerless (Mardin, 1986) and so their viewpoint can be ignored. Nevertheless, there is an increasing emphasis on the need for assessments of the structure, process and outcomes of health care systems (Donabedian, 1966) and for such assessments to consider the patients' perspective. Medical care should be efficient, cost-effective and appropriate: it should also be accessible and acceptable to patients (Hopkins, 1990).

In the UK and elsewhere, quality assessment is now seen as an important approach to raising standards of care and increasing the accountability of the providers of care (Hughes and Humphrey, 1990). A central proposal of recent Government publications in the UK is that doctors should assess the quality of the care they provide through regular, systematic medical audit, in which surveys of patients' views and experiences represent a major area of activity. While there are a number of conceptual and methodological difficulties in assessing patients' satisfaction with care, it nevertheless represents an important outcome measure, and enables choices to be made between alternative methods of organising and providing health care (Fitzpatrick, 1990). At Walton Hospital, we are currently working on a study of patients' experiences of services for epilepsy and their satisfaction with those services; and we know of similar work which is being undertaken in The Netherlands (Suurmeijer, 1991). Here again is an area where the validation of global outcomes are urgently required.

REFERENCES

Baker GA, Smith DF, Dewey M, et al (1991) The development of a seizure severity scale as an outcome measure in epilepsy. Epilepsy Res. 8:245–251.

Cartwright A (1983) Health surveys; in practice and in potential. London King Edward's Hospital Fund.

Cramer JA, Smith DB, Mattson RH et al (1983) A method of quantification for the evaluation of anti-epileptic drug therapy. Neurology (Cleveland); 33 (Suppl 1):26–37.

Donabedian A (1966) Evaluating the quality of medical care. Millbank Memorial Fund Quarterly 44; 166–206.

Drummond MF (1987) Resource allocation; decisions in health care: a role for quality of life assessments. Journal of Chronic Diseases; 40:605–616.

Fitzpatrick R (1990) Surveys of patient satisfaction. Important general considerations. BMJ; 302:887–9.

Hopkins A (1990) Measuring the quality of medical care. London: Royal College of Physicians.

Hughes J and Humphrey C (1990) Medical Audit in General Practice. London: King's Fund Centre.

Jacoby A (1992) Epilepsy and the quality of everyday life. Social Science and Medicine; 34:657–666.

Jacoby A, Johnson A, Chadwick DW (1992) The psychosocial outcomes of antiepileptic drug withdrawal. Epilepsia; 33:1023–1032.

Mardin EM (1986) Consumer evaluation of human services. Social Policy and Administration; 20:185–199.

Mattson RH, Cramer JA, Collins JF et al (1985). Comparison of carbamazepine, phenobarbital, phenytoin and primidone in partial and secondary generalised tonic-clonic seizures. New Eng. J. of Med.; 313: 145–151.

Meador KJ, Loring DW, Allen ME et al (1991) Comparative cognitive effects of carbamazepine and phenytoin in healthy adults. Neurology; 41:1537–1540.

Scambler G (1989) Epilepsy: the experience of illness. Tavistock, Routledge, London.

Slevin MI, Plant H, Lynch D et al (1987) Who should measure quality of life, doctor or patient? Br. J. Cancer; 57:109–112.

Smith DF, Baker GA, Dewey M et al (1991) Seizure frequency, patient-perceived seizure severity and the psychosocial consequences of intractable epilepsy. Epilepsy Res. 9:231–241.

Suurmeijer TP (1991) Quality of care: perceptions of patients. Paper presented at 19th International Epilepsy Congress, Rio de Janeiro, Brazil.

Turnbull DM, Howell D, Rawlins MD and Chadwick DW (1985) Which drug for the adult epileptic patient: phenytoin or valproate? B.M.J. 290:815–819.

Van Belle G. & Temkin N. (1981) Design strategies in the clinical evaluation of new antiepileptic drugs. In: Recent Advances in Epilepsy 1, Eds. Pedley T.A. & Meldrum B.S., Churchill Livingstone, Ed. Lon. Mel. N.Y. 93–111.

Ziller RC (1974) Self-other orientations and quality of life. Social Indications Research; 1:301–327.

HEALTH-RELATED QUALITY OF LIFE

Bert Spilker, Ph.D., M.D.

Executive Director
Orphan Medical
13911 Ridgedale Drive
Minnetonka, Minnesota 55305, U.S.A.

INTRODUCTION

Two Aspects of Quality of Life

This chapter provides an overview of the nature and status of quality of life evaluations of new medicines and other treatments in clinical trials. There are two major aspects of quality of life: The environmental aspect of quality of life and health-related quality of life. The environmental aspect of quality of life is often evaluated by organizations outside the medical field. The components they often consider for different locations or areas include (1) air quality, (2) water quality, (3) school quality, (4) population density, (5) cultural opportunities, (6) social/economic status, and (7) community spirit. On the other hand, health-related quality of life encompasses a number of distinct domains related to patients and their well-being. The individual components of quality of life are discussed in a few (three to six) broad domains (i.e., categories). In this chapter, four domains are described: (1) physical abilities/capabilities, (2) psychological status, (3 social status, and (4) economic status/employment. Although health-related quality of life relates mainly to individual patients and groups of patients, it also may be applied, as can environment-related quality of life, to individual communities, regions, or nations. In the remainder of this chapter the term quality of life refers only to health-related quality of life.

Levels of Quality of Life

The various levels of health-related quality of life may be viewed as a pyramid (Figure 1). Of the three levels of quality of life illustrated in Figure 1, the most inclusive

Quantitative Assessment in Epilepsy Care, Edited by H. Meinardi et al.
Plenum Press, New York, 1993

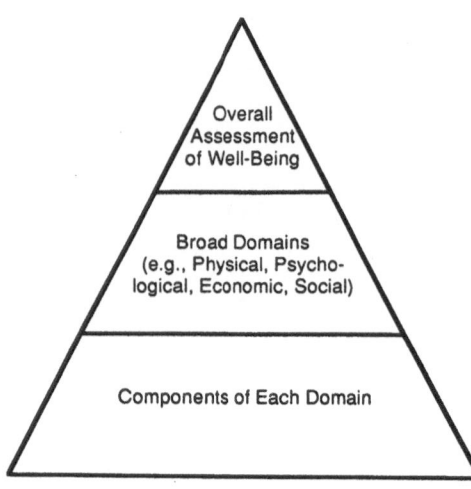

Figure 1. Three levels of quality of life assessments. Reprinted from B. Spilker "Introduction," *Quality of Life Assessments in Clinical Trials* (ed. B. Spilker), Raven Press, New York, 1990, pp. 3–9, with permission.

is that of overall assessment of patient well-being. This is evaluated in clinical trials by asking patients a question such as: "Overall how would you assess your well-being today?" Alternatively, one could ask "How would you assess your overall well-being since you began this trial, or compared with the start of this trial?." This question has often been asked in clinical trials as a "global assessment" of the patient's well-being, even before the question was referred to as a quality of life assessment. The second level relates to the four broad domains described above—physical, psychological, social, and economic. The third and most broad level of quality of life consists of the individual components of each domain. Each domain has many components or aspects. Physical well-being or physical status is made up of many separate physical abilities. Psychological status is made up of cognitive function, depression, anxiety, etc. The other two domains likewise are made up of separate components. Each of the components of the domains may be measured with separate scales or may be measured along with other components using a single scale.

The Filtering Phenomenon

To understand why patients who experience the same general benefits and adverse reactions as other patients assess their quality of life differently, it is necessary to examine Figure 2. This figure illustrates that the various safety measures, efficacy measures, and additional factors such as treatment convenience and cost are all summed up by patients and are, in a sense, filtered through the patients' values, beliefs, and judgments, finally becoming integrated in an overall assessment by that individual. This overall assessment is in terms of physical status and ability, psychological well-being, social interactions and economic status—i.e., their quality of life. It is apparent that some patients are hardly bothered by severe adverse reactions whereas other patients are bothered to a far greater degree by less severe adverse reactions of the same type. Some patients may focus so much on the cost of a treatment that their

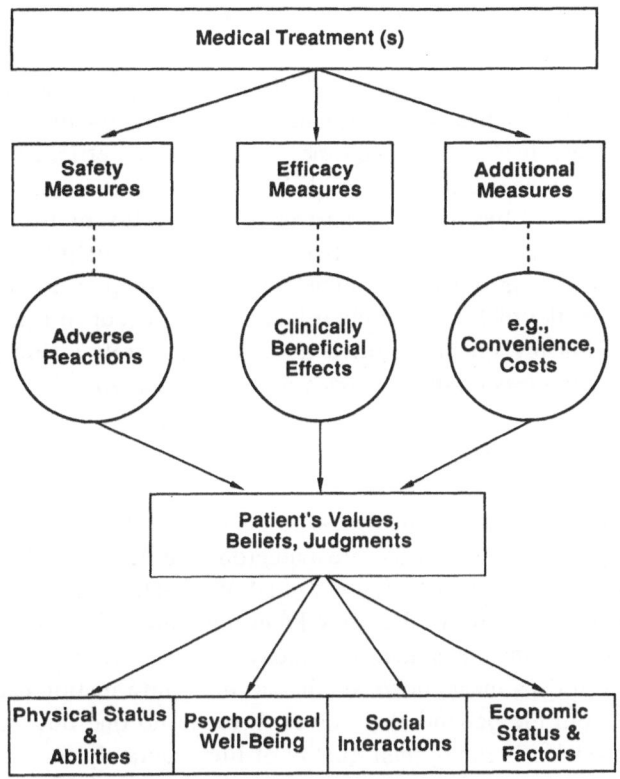

Figure 2. Model of how clinical aspects of efficacy (i.e., benefits), safety (e.g., adverse reactions) or other factors filter through the patient's values and beliefs to influence the domains of his or her quality of life. Reprinted from B. Spilker "Introduction," in *Quality of Life Assessments in Clinical Trials* (ed. B. Spilker), Raven Press, New York, 1990, pp. 3–9, with permission.

judgment of quality of life is made independent of the treatment's benefits or even adverse reactions. Values, beliefs, and judgments are those aspects of a patient's being that integrate dissimilar effects of efficacy, safety, cost, convenience, and other factors and allow the individual to arrive at an overall judgment of quality of life. These summary judgments are, thus, based on all three levels of the pyramid.

The quality of life of patients in a clinical trial may be assessed for individuals, groups of patients, or in terms of large patient populations either within or outside of clinical trials.

ISSUES

A number of issues are described below that relate to current controversies and debates within the field of quality of life assessment. Not all of these issues are controversial.

Quality of Life as a Surrogate Endpoint, as "Soft" versus "Hard" Endpoints, or as a Fad

It is sometimes suggested that quality of life is a surrogate endpoint in clinical trials. This is not true. Quality of life is the ultimate goal of therapy—to improve how patients feel, think, and behave. It is an important measure of clinical efficacy.

The issue is also raised as to whether quality of life measures are "soft" (i.e., subjective) or somewhat more objective. The answer is that quality of life endpoints are soft. There are no reliable "hard" (i.e., objective) measures of quality of life. Nonetheless, quality of life is not a surrogate for something else. Another frequently raised issue concerns whether quality of life is merely a fad, (fads do occur in science and in clinical medicine). Unquestionably, quality of life is not a fad, or merely fashionable at the current time. It is the ultimate measure of a patient's reaction to therapy.

Who Assesses Quality of Life?

Can physicians and spouses reliably assess quality of life of patients? The answer to this question is absolutely not. There are numerous studies that all point to the same conclusion. Spouses and physicians may not reliably predict the answers to quality of life questions for patients, even those that they know intimately. This does not mean that a spouse or physician cannot understand accurately how another person judges his or her own quality of life. It does mean, however, that accurate information can only be obtained in a clinical trial from the patients themselves, because no one but the patients know if their spouse or physician is rating their quality of life accurately.

When Should Quality of Life Be Measured?

During what phase of clinical drug development should quality of life be measured? Most quality of life trials are conducted during Phases III and IV. The parameters that are going to be particularly important to measure are often identified during Phase II clinical trials. In addition, it is important that quality of life data be available for a sponsor to use prior to the initial marketing of a medicine. This means that the data should be collected during Phase III (usually Phase IIIb—i.e., after the dossier for registration is submitted) so that it can be used prior to marketing or at the time of initial marketing in promotions and in presentation to different formulary committees.

Should Quality of Life Be Evaluated for All Medicines?

Whether quality of life should be studied for all medicines has been widely discussed. In most people's view, it is not necessary to conduct quality of life trials for many new investigational medicines. Some examples where quality of life trials are important are when there are a number of medicines of different types competing in the same disease area. Such trials may be important where there are numerous "me-too" medicines and a sponsor is attempting to differentiate its medicine from the others. Finally, quality of life trials are valuable in those therapeutic areas where quality of life data may help speed regulatory approval. The therapeutic area in which this is most important is oncology. It is believed that quality of life data may help in the approval of new oncologic agents, particularly if improvements are noteworthy in quality of life. Quality of life data have not been the sole determinant for the approval of any investigational medicine. However, such data may support a medicine's approval.

How Are Quality of Life Data Used?

Quality of life data may be used by health planners to allocate health care resources, particularly those of various governments. Formulary committees are using quality of life data to decide whether to put medicines onto their formularies. They often debate differences in quality of life data as a basis for whether or not to accept new medicines onto formularies. Physicians use quality of life data to help choose medicines for their patients.

General versus Specific Scales of Quality of Life

In considering disease-specific versus general scales, it is important to realize that there are only a few diseases for which quality of life scales that are validated and useful, have been generated. The majority of diseases do not have such scales, and trials must rely on data obtained with general scales. In addition to specific scales relating to a disease, there are a number of specific scales relating to a patient's function, such as sexual function and emotional function. Another specific scale would be one relating to a specific population (e.g. a geriatric population).

Use of a Single Index versus a Battery of Tests

A single index of quality of life or a battery of tests can be used in a clinical trial. A single index refers to a single scale that measures multiple domains and components of those domains. A battery involves multiple tests, each one of which will measure one or more components of a domain; in some cases, a test could measure two different domains and then be combined with other tests to create a battery covering the entire scope of domains being evaluated.

Alternatives when No Disease-Specific Scale Exists

At the present time there are no well-validated quality of life tests or measures in the field of epilepsy. This is not unique or even unusual in medicine, because only about a dozen diseases have well-validated quality of life tests. When no disease-specific measures (i.e., instrument) exists, a sponsor may choose to use a general validated instrument, such as the SIP (Sickness Impact Profile) which has been validated in many different diseases and in many different patient populations. A second approach is to use a battery of validated instruments if no disease-specific measure exists.

A third possibility is to ask three to six (or more) disease-specific questions at the end and possibly at other points in the clinical trial. These questions should address the most important quality of life issues in that disease that are not covered by general instruments. Such questions should not be used as a substitute for a validated general quality of life index scale, or battery of instruments, but as a supplement. Neither should these questions be referred to as an instrument. They may be questions that patients answer themselves using a Likert scale, or they may be questions in which the investigator or administrator of the quality of life test records how a patient responds to the questions. One question relating to epilepsy might be "Are your seizures more or less intense (severe) since you started in this trial?" A visual analog scale could be used to assess this parameter; it could be graded from "much more intense," to "no seizures have occurred." These two ends are called anchors of the visual analog scale. A Likert scale should have at least five and possibly seven categories, such as (1) the worst they have ever been, (2) much worse, (3) slightly worse, (4) about the same, (5) slightly better, (6) much better, and (7) no seizures have occurred.

Another question might be, "To what degree have your seizures affected your ability to function at the level you desire since you started in this trial?" For this question one could use a visual analog scale graded from "cannot function at all," at one end to, "best level I have ever experienced," at the other end of the scale. Data from these questions may be statistically analyzed from each treatment group, clinically interpreted, and used appropriately for various purposes. These purposes could include registration of a medicine as well as promotion. Using patient response to a question about severity of seizures could lead to problems such as one patient not feeling that his quality of life was improved as a result of less severe seizures, because the number was unaltered. Some patients also may not feel that their quality of life was improved if the intensity of seizures was decreased but their duration or number was increased.

One caution about using individual questions rather than a prepared and tested instrument (scale) to obtain data about quality of life is that the data from the questions should not be combined in any way or the questions themselves referred to as an instrument or scale. If the questions are referred to as a scale it will invite strong criticism from experts challenging the results and questioning the validity of the so-called scale. Those challenges would have merit in that the combined questions would not have been validated by the authors. Nonetheless, the data obtained with individual questions can be used (without being combined) as relevant assessments of pertinent quality of life issues.

Control Groups

In quality of life trials the issue often arises as to whether patients should be "controlled" by (1) using a concomitant control group, (2) having patients serving as their own control, or (3) using historical controls. The time of assessment must also be decided and indicated in the protocol, so that each investigator assesses the same time period in measuring quality of life. Possibilities include (1) the immediate present, (2) the last 24 hours, (3) the last week, or (4) since the patient's last visit to the clinic. Of course, all clinical trial protocols should indicate the period to be considered for a patient's assessment, particularly for adverse reactions, but also for other safety and efficacy measures.

Measuring Events versus the Patient's Assessment of Those Events

In determining whether one should quantitate (i.e., measure or count) events or one should assess how patients value those events, it is important to understand the nature of the trial and how each of those events might be important. On the other hand, if one is quantitating events such as the number of transfusion of blood, it is less relevant to quality of life than the assessment of how patients value those events. For example, many children do not mind visits to hospitals more frequently to treat their asthma if they are allowed to be more free and engage in more activities between their visits to the hospital. They may feel that their quality of life has increased, even though their number of hospital visits has also increased.

Measuring Abilities versus Capabilities

Finally, it is important to consider whether one should measure patient activities—that is, what they actually do—versus capabilities, i.e., what the patients *can* do. There is a strong case that can be made for both of these assessments; the choice must be made for each individual trial.

MISUSE OF QUALITY OF LIFE TRIALS

Unfortunately, the number and choice of domains and components of each domain to study in a clinical trial often are decided a priori based on what the sponsor wants to demonstrate as an outcome of the trial. This is the approach that is commonly followed—but is it acceptable? In the overall area of clinical trials it is not generally acceptable to tailor the design of a trial to obtain the results one wishes to achieve. For example, does one tailor Phase II or III trials to demonstrate a preconceived outcome? This question should cause medical professionals to raise their eyebrows, because specific Phase II and III trial results are not specifically known in advance. The very purpose of conducting a clinical trial is to determine the outcome.

How are Quality of Life Trials Misused?

There are three common ways in which quality of life trials are misused.

(1) By working backward from the specific end result that the protocol planners expect to observe to choose the test or tests which will demonstrate this result most convincingly.

(2) By choosing the most toxic or inactive comparative treatment or treatments.

(3) By using a large number of instruments, and selecting only some of the results to present in reports or publications.

PROPER USE OF QUALITY OF LIFE TRIALS

Quality of life trials therefore, often stack the desk in favour of the preferred treatment. This is not an appropriate means to design or conduct quality of life trials. Can a more objective approach be found? The answer to this question is yes. **The most objective approach to conducting quality of life trials is to evaluate all domains. Multiple components of each domain should be assessed in all quality of life trials.**

How will assessing all domains help various groups who are concerned with quality of life data? **Sponsors** will know that their competitors will not unfairly test and malign their medicines. **Formulary committees** will know that quality of life data submitted to their groups are more objective and fair. **Physicians** will know that the data and advertisements they review are more balanced and credible. **Patients** will receive more appropriate treatment because of the better information received, and better decisions made, by their physicians. **Regulators** will note improved standards in this area, and they will receive more objective quality of life data from sponsors on new investigational medicines.

Why should sponsors adopt this practice? Because the consequences of not adopting this practice are that quality of life trials will obtain a reputation of being biased and unreliable. As a result, quality of life trials will not be useful for their current purposes.

The pressures to implement this concept should come in future from (1) journal editors, (2) formulary committees, (3) regulatory authorities, 4) ethics committees or institutional review boards, (5) and enlightened pharmaceutical industry personnel.

Undoubtedly, this approach will generate a large quantity of negative (i.e., no effect) data. But everyone will be assured that authors are not committing the sins of omission (i.e., not studying areas where important results could be found). People in all therapeutic areas will no longer have to wonder if important results were missed or avoided that would have been obtained by a more complete and honest evaluation of quality of life.

In conclusion, the most important points to consider in assessing quality of life are: (1) that validated scales must be used in clinical trials if the data are to be believed and accepted by various groups, and (2) that the standards used in quality of life trials must be as high as those in other well controlled clinical trials. Unless standards of quality of life trials improve, the data obtained will be seriously questioned and viewed as unreliable.

THE QUALITY OF LIFE OF PATIENTS WITH EPILEPSY

Dave Smith, M.D., M.R.C.P.[1]
and Gus Baker, Ph.D., B.A., M.Clin.Psychol., A.F.B.Ps.[2]

[1]Lecturer in Neurology
[2]Principal Clinical Neuropsychologist
Department of Neurosciences
University of Liverpool
Walton Hospital
Liverpool, United Kingdom

INTRODUCTION

Epilepsy is a common condition with a prevalence of 6/1000 and a life-time cumulative incidence of 3% (Hauser & Kurland 1975). The overall prognosis is good (Annegers et al 1979) but 25–40% of patients continue to have frequent seizures despite optimal doses of conventional drugs (AEDs). This group of patients, approximately 100,000 in the UK, have little chance of spontaneous remission (Elwes et al 1984), are often exposed to high doses of toxic medication and, despite no obvious physical deficit, are often socially and psychologically handicapped.

Surgical treatment (Engel 1987) produces relief of seizures in a selected minority but for most of these patients the only hope is the development of more effective, less toxic new AEDs (Meldrum & Porter 1986). The need for new drugs and more sensitive methods of assessing their efficacy (Van Belle & Temkin 1981) are well recognised. This latter issue is especially relevant where remission of seizures is unlikely and where reduction of seizure severity or improvement in psychological well-being, with a consequent improvement in quality of life, may be more realistic therapeutic goals. Quality of life has been suggested as an alternative outcome measure for the assessment of both medical (Van Belle & Temkin 1981) and surgical treatment (Hauser 1987) but the development of a satisfactory instrument has been hampered by the prevalent belief that such measures provide unreliable data. However there is increasing evidence that health-related quality of life (HRQL) instruments are useful indicators of medical outcome (Spilker 1990).

Quantitative Assessment in Epilepsy Care, Edited by H. Meinardi et al.
Plenum Press, New York, 1993

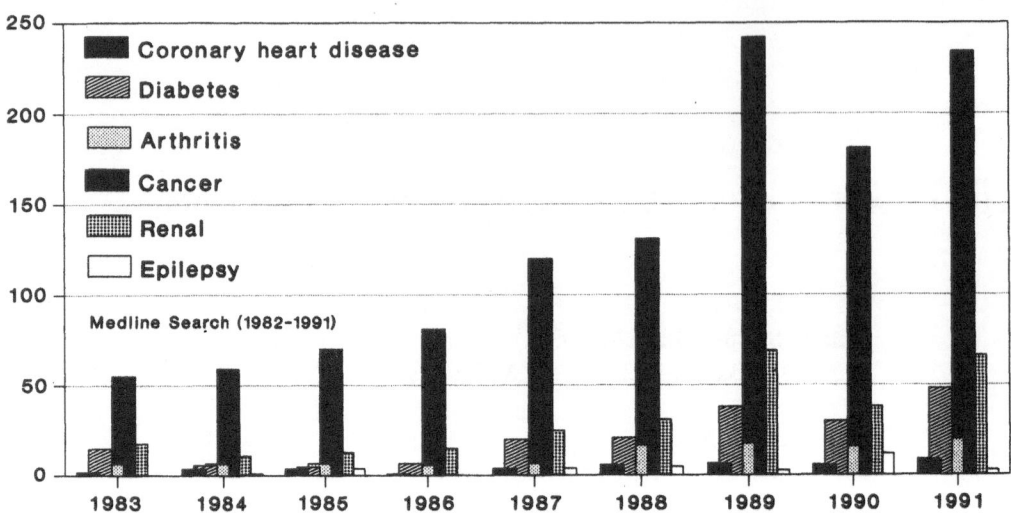

Figure 1. Trends in quality of life research for chronic conditions.

Measures of HRQL should consider the impact of a condition, and its treatment, on physical, social and psychological well-being. Whilst generic instruments may be useful for the allocation of health care resources (Drummond 1987), disease-specific (DSQL) instruments are most appropriate for assessing treatment effects in clinical trials (Guyatt et al 1989) and it is generally agreed that HRQL measures should concentrate on individual patient perception (Schipper et al 1990). DSQL instruments have been developed for several common conditions but, in comparison to other more "fashionable" chronic illnesses, epilepsy has, until recently, received limited attention in HRQL research (fig.1).

The Psychosocial Prognosis of Epilepsy and Quality of Life

A dearth of systematic, population-based studies (Zielinski 1986) precludes accurate estimation of the incidence/prevalence of the secondary problems associated with epilepsy. However evidence from "biased," hospital-based statistics suggests that the medical prognosis is closely related to the psychosocial prognosis and, hence, to the patients' quality of life.

Whilst patients with well-controlled epilepsy experience few problems (Trostle et al 1989, Jacoby et al 1992), those with refractory seizures are susceptible to a constellation of physical risks, social restrictions and psychological consequences which may be more disabling than the seizures themselves (Commission 1978).

The aetiology of the psychopathology associated with intractable epilepsy has not been satisfactorily investigated (Whitman & Hermann 1989)—the biomedical model is inadequate (Engel 1977) and a multietiological model, emphasizing the importance of social variables (Hermann & Whitman 1986) is more appropriate.

Goodyer (1988) defines a social withdrawal syndrome with several contributory factors. The high level of unemployment (Elwes et al 1991) may be attributable to a lack of formal qualifications (Harrison & Taylor 1976), legislative restrictions (Craig & Oxley 1988), perceived stigma (Scambler 1989), seizure frequency (Scambler & Hopkins 1980) and, possibly, subtle impairment of visuo-spatial and motor performance (Batzell et al 1980). Low rates of marriage (Dansky et al 1980) can be explained by limited social contacts (Mittan 1986), low levels of self-esteem (Arnston et al 1986), lack of financial resources (Thompson & Oxley 1988) and hyposexuality in males (Toone et al 1980).

Abbey & Andrews (1985) identified the main psychological determinants of life quality to be self-esteem, internal locus of control and the absence of anxiety and depression, all of which can be adversely affected by epilepsy. Anxiety, which is the commonest disturbance of mood in patients with epilepsy (Betts 1981), can be explained by the unpredictability (Smith et al 1991) and fear of seizures (Mittan 1986), fear of exposure of epilepsy (Scambler 1989) and external locus of control (Arnston et al 1986). Depression may be a consequence of protracted, unrelieved anxiety (Hermann 1979), social isolation or chronic administration of sedative AEDs, particularly phenobarbitone (Robertson et al 1987). Low self-esteem in adults (Arnston et al 1986) may be due to chronic unemployment, single status and perceived stigma (Scambler 1989) whilst in children (Matthews et al 1982), it is the product of negative peer reactions and parental overprotectiveness (Bagley 1971). Feelings of loss of control are understandable because of dependence on medication prescribed by others, restriction of activities and opportunities imposed by others and by the unpredictability of the seizures themselves.

Smith et al (1991) indicate that psychological problems are associated with each other while overall psychological well-being has been related to "self-image discrepancy" (Collings 1990), multiple seizure types (Hermann et al 1982), financial stress and the number of major life events in the previous year (Hermann et al 1990). Conversely it is likely that seizure control, although clearly dependent on several biological factors not amenable to change, may be influenced by significant life events (Webster & Mawer 1989) or stress (Temkin & Davis 1984) and that mood, or change in mood, could influence patient perception of seizure severity.

Measurement of Quality of Life in Patients with Epilepsy

Clearly the interaction between the physical, social and psychological manifestations of epilepsy is complex which might explain why no comprehensive quality of life model for epilepsy has been developed.

However quality of life research in epilepsy has gained impetus in the last few years. Cross-sectional studies have been conducted in patients well controlled (Jacoby 1992, Jacoby et al 1992) and chronic epilepsy (Collings 1990). Furthermore HRQL has been used in the assessment of the efficacy of both medical (Smith et al 1992) and surgical treatment (Vickrey et al 1992) of refractory epilepsy. The topical nature of this subject is indicated by the inclusion of seminars dedicated to quality of life in epilepsy in the 19th World Congress on Epilepsy, the 2nd Palm Desert Conference on the Surgical Treatment of the Epilepsies, and the recent European Epilepsy Conference.

The remainder of this article concentrates on published research dealing with measurement of QOL in patients with epilepsy. However two instruments, neither of which can be considered to be QOL measures in their own right, deserve attention because they have the potential for inclusion in comprehensive HRQL instruments.

The Washington Psychosocial Seizure Inventory (WPSI)

The WPSI (Dodrill et al 1980) considers adjustment to epilepsy in 8 domains: family background, emotional adjustment, vocational adjustment, financial status, adjustment to seizures, medical management and overall psychosocial function. The score in each domain places an individual in one of four categories of adjustment (fig. 2).

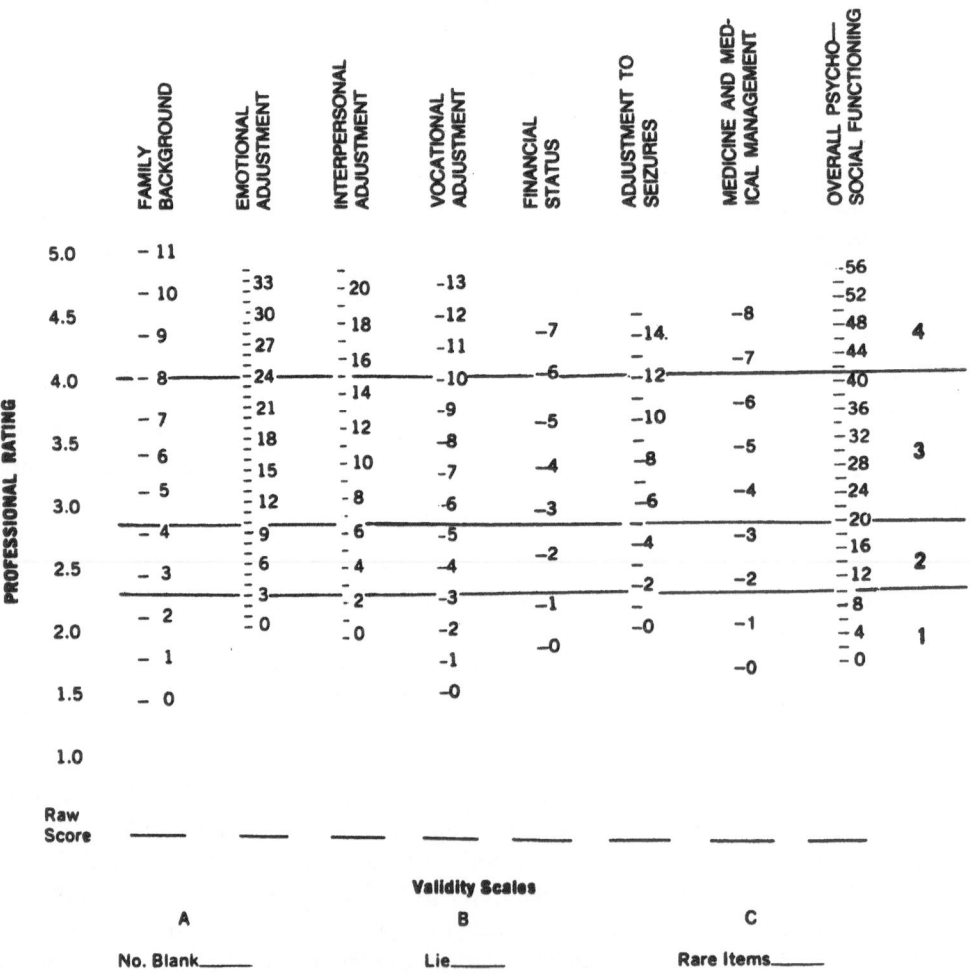

Figure 2. Washington psychosocial seizure inventory profile form (©Carl B. Dodrill, 1978).

Inter-rater reliability is high (Pearsons correlation coefficient (PCC) 0.80–0.95), there are significant correlations between patient and professional ratings for each scale, test-retest reliability (PCC 0.66–0.87) and internal consistency (alpha 0.68–0.95) are acceptable. The scales are independent but there is a high degree of correlation (PCC 0.48–0.93) between the base scales and the overall psychosocial function scale. This instrument has been further developed by the original research team and used extensively by other investigators.

Batzel et al (1980) demonstrated that the Vocational Adjustment Scale (VAS) of the WPSI was the most important of two independently significant predictors of employment status thus providing evidence for the construct validity of this scale.

Dodrill et al (1984a) found levels of overall psychosocial dysfunction which were similar to clinically derived estimates (Rodin et al 1977) suggesting that the WPSI is capable of defining the prevalence of psychosocial problems in patients with active epilepsy. Furthermore Trostle et al (1989) demonstrated significantly better adjustment in white, middle-class patients with well-controlled epilepsy than that observed in clinic-based samples (Dodrill et al 1984a). Patients in the Rochester group (Trostle et al 1989) with continuing seizures, despite antiepileptic drug therapy, had profiles similar to the other groups (Dodrill et al 1984a). Thus the WPSI appears to differentiate between populations who would be predicted to have different levels of psychosocial adjustment lending support to its discriminant construct validity. The WPSI has been used in the assessment of AED effects (Wilensky et al 1983), to measure the outcome of counselling (Earl 1986) and behavioral therapy (Tan & Bruni 1986). It is now widely used as a measure of post-operative psychosocial adjustment in many epilepsy surgery centres in the USA. Thus the conclusion from the initial publication that: "the WPSI is an objective indicator of psychosocial adjustment with several potential research and clinical applications" (Dodrill et al 1980) has proved, at least in the USA, to be correct.

Major criticisms include the use of professional opinion to determine the original item pool (Trostle et al 1989) and the use of purely statistical methods to separate items into sub-scales (Vickrey et al 1992). However the main barrier to this instruments world-wide acceptance is its application in non-US populations. Dodrill et al (1984b) compared and conceded that the WPSI may be insensitive to cultural differences to the extent that figures in countries other than the USA may be under-estimates. No satisfactory attempt has been made to standardize this instrument outside the USA but the WPSI, or some of its elements, could clearly be incorporated into QOL measures for epilepsy.

The Epilepsy Social Effects Scale

Chaplin et al (1990) describe a scale whose content was derived from patient-generated statements which were categorised, by professionals, into 21 areas of concern. The measure is complicated by the inclusion of a professional-based weighting system of doubtful validity. Content validity can be assumed, but "criterion-related validity" is not established and test-retest reliability (PCC 0.50–0.75, mean 0.64) of the 14 validated areas (Table 1) is barely acceptable.

Table 1. Pearson's correlational analysis

Validated Areas of Concern	Correlation Coefficients	Validated Areas of Concern	Correlation Coefficients
(1) Attacks	0.72	(13) Life	0.73
(3) Seizures	0.62	(14) Family	0.51
(4) Employment	0.72	(15) Medication	0.53
(5) The future	0.37	(16) Medical profession	0.71
(10) Travel	0.50	(18) Emotional reaction	0.73
(11) Social life	0.67	(19) Social isolation	0.71
(12) Leisure	0.62	(20) Energy	0.75

The scale was administered to 192 patients with a recent diagnosis of epilepsy (within previous 36 months) (Chaplin et al 1992). Most common problem areas were acceptance of diagnosis (64%), fear of having seizures (80%) and fear of stigma affecting employment (69%). Severe problems occurred in > 10% of patients in only 4 areas; fear of having seizures, fear of stigma affecting employment, adverse affects on leisure pursuits and lack of energy. The number and severity of problems were significantly greater in those who had experienced > 4 seizures and in those with seizures during previous 12 months. The authors conclude that the psychosocial effects are more closely related to the severity of the condition than the label itself whilst conceding that this label is more evident in those with persistent seizures.

This is a promising measure but examination of its factorial structure and better evidence of reliability, particularly internal consistency, and validity is required. Overall this scale has potential as a measure of social adjustment and, with development, could be included in a HRQL model for epilepsy.

Quality of Life in Newly Diagnosed Epilepsy

The impact of epilepsy on the QOL of a homogenous group of newly diagnosed patients has not been investigated. This will largely be determined by the initial response to treatment, the socio-economic implications of the diagnosis per se and individual psychosocial adjustment which, in turn, depends on innate coping resources and social support. The heterogeneity of the population described by Chaplin et al (1992) precludes useful comment on this subject. However the psychosocial impact of diagnosis, and treatment, should be clarified in the forthcoming prospective study of immediate versus delayed treatment in patients with a single seizure or early epilepsy.

Quality of Life of Epilepsy in Remission

The work of Ann Jacoby (Jacoby 1992, Jacoby et al 1992), under the auspices of the MRC Antiepileptic Drug Withdrawal Study, merits considerable attention. In the first study (Jacoby 1992) she administered a QOL questionnaire which combined pre-coded and open-ended questions with previously validated measures of perceived health status, affect, self-esteem, mastery and stigma to 607 patients of whom 71% were in remission of at least 2 years.

Overall, reported levels of distress were low, participants were well adjusted and experienced few problems. Objective evidence for this is indicated by the high levels of employment, marriage and their active social lives. For the majority of patients every day quality of life was not impaired and this was attributed to their seizure-free status. The period seizure-free was significantly associated with the extent to which patients worried about epilepsy, self-assessed health status, whether they felt social activities were restricted or they did not do things because of epilepsy and whether they felt epilepsy made it more difficult to get a job. A minority of patients experienced significant problems. The extent to which they worried about their epilepsy was directly related to stigma and emotional well-being independent of the period seizure-free. The author suggests that adjustment to epilepsy is dependent not only on clinical course but also on innate psychological coping resources. Self-esteem and mastery were inversely related to expressed levels of anxiety in those patients whose epilepsy is in remission but not for those in whom epilepsy was classified as active, i.e. seizures within previous two years. She contends that in patients with active epilepsy seizure activity determines these parameters whilst for those in remission adjustment may be more important. A significant flaw of this otherwise excellent study was the lack of multivariate analysis which would have permitted testing of both these hypotheses using the data collected.

In the second study (Jacoby et al 1992) the same questionnaire was administered to 468 patients 2 years after randomisation. 42% of those randomised to slow withdrawal and 19% continuing medication had experienced recurrence of seizures. As expected, in each treatment group, the psychosocial profile was better in those remaining seizure-free. Interestingly, relapse on medication was associated with more distress than relapse associated with planned withdrawal. The authors conclude that for those patients with a low risk of relapse the benefits of AED withdrawal may be considerable. However, the implications of relapse may be devastating and the decision to withdraw therapy should be made in the light of each individual psychological and social circumstances.

QUALITY OF LIFE OF PATIENTS WITH CHRONIC EPILEPSY

QOL of Individuals with Chronic Epilepsy

Kendrick & Trimble (1992) have assessed QOL in 50 residents at the Chalfont Centre for Epilepsy. Patients were asked to identify specific areas of importance in five key domains: physical functioning, cognitive state, emotional status, social functioning and economic/employment status. They rated the severity of each problem and their own quality of life, for each area, relative to their associates. This allowed the generation of values for the difference between actual (NOW) and desired (LIKE) QOL (the N–L distance) which can be portrayed as a composite score or as an individual profile. This highly individualised approach is consistent with the gap hypothesis of QOL (Calman 1984). Whilst this method is interesting it involves repeated interviews conducted by trained investigators. Therefore, it may be a useful technique for identifying specific problems in individuals but, in its current form, could not be applied to large scale clinical trials. However this approach may be usefully applied in the assessment of epilepsy surgery where the patient identifies specific target outcomes (Taylor 1993).

QOL of Community–Based Patients with Epilepsy

Collings (1990) examined well being in a community based sample (n = 392) of patients with active epilepsy. A questionnaire containing 6 well-being scales (self-esteem, life fulfilment, social and inter-personal difficulties, general physical health, worries and affect balance), 10 epilepsy related and 8 socio-demographic variables was administered. Factor analysis permitted the total scores of the six well being scales to be combined to form an "overall well-being scale." Univariate analysis revealed that overall well-being was significantly related to self-image discrepancy, time since diagnosis, seizure frequency, certainty of diagnosis, absence seizures and full time employment. However multivariate analysis demonstrated that self-image discrepancy alone accounted for 56% of the variance of well-being. Thus the discrepancy between current self perception and anticipated self without epilepsy was the best predictor of overall well being. The author suggests that this may be attributable to "the interaction between the environment in which the person has developed psychologically and the stigma of having epilepsy" or to individual misconceptions about the condition. Uncertainty about the diagnosis and the recent onset of epilepsy were associated with low well being possibly reflecting the stress encountered due to a perceived lack of control over their condition. Not surprisingly, seizure frequency was directly related to well being whilst those with absence seizures fared well. These issues probably relate to the visibility of an individual's epilepsy.

The author emphasises that when assessing quality of life, patients' perception of themselves and their circumstances are as important as biological and socio-demographic factors.

Quality of Life as an Outcome Measure in Epilepsy

Assessment of treatment effects in chronic epilepsy has been based, almost entirely, on physicians judgements about change in seizure frequency attributable to treatment intervention. This has never been appropriate and is no longer acceptable.

Temporal lobe surgery is highly effective in selected patients but induction of seizure freedom is no guarantee of long-term psychosocial benefit. The converse is also true i.e. patients with continuing auras and infrequent complex partial seizures are not seizure free but may consider themselves to be significantly improved. The patient has to decide if remission, or reduction, of seizures outweighs any unexpected fixed physical deficit or poorer than expected psychosocial adaptation.

The situation is equally complex when one considers the assessment of the efficacy of new antiepileptic drugs in clinical trials. There is little doubt that some of the new drugs are well tolerated and diminish seizure frequency but few, if any, patients achieve protracted remission. The issue for those patients who complete AED trials is whether or not any beneficial treatment effects outweigh the adverse effects caused by the increased anticonvulsant burden. In either case the patient is required to make a judgement regarding change in health status or health-related quality of life attributable to treatment. Neither temporal lobe surgery programmes nor conventional AED trials are capable of measuring this. However significant advances in both areas have recently been made.

Temporal Lobe Surgery and HRQL

The aims of surgery for epilepsy are the abolition of seizures and improvement of quality of life. Whilst the former is easily observable the latter is unpredictable. In response to the National Institutes of Health (1990) recommendation that an HRQL measure should be developed to assess the effectiveness of epilepsy surgery programmes, the UCLA group (Vickrey et al 1992) have created such an instrument.

The epilepsy surgery inventory (ESI-55) is the combination of a previously validated measure, the SF36 (Ware and Sherbourne 1992) and 19 epilepsy-specific items. The instrument considers 11 domains of quality of life; health perceptions, energy/fatigue, overall QOL, social function, emotional well-being, cognitive function, physical function, pain, role limitations due to emotional, physical and memory problems and a single item reflecting change in health status.

A postal questionnaire including the ESI-55, a mood profile (Thayer 1967) and questions regarding seizure status and medication was completed by 200 patients who had received, or been evaluated for epilepsy surgery. Post-operative seizure classification (n = 142) was simple; patients with no seizures (seizure free), patients with simple partial seizures only (auras), patients with complex partial or secondary generalised tonic-clonic seizures (seizures).

This first evaluation of the ESI-55 reveals excellent psychometric properties. Ten out of the 11 scales had an alpha score of > 0.70 indicating acceptable reliability for use in clinical trials. Simple factor analysis produced a three factor solution; mental health, physical health and cognitive functions/role limitations on to which all scales were highly loaded. Notably global QOL was loaded onto the mental health factor. Correlational analyses with the mood profile demonstrate both convergent and discriminate construct validity. The most notable finding was the ability of the scales to differentiate between patients according to the very simple seizure classification. Seizure-free patients scored higher than those with continuing seizures on all 11 scales (p ≤ 0.05). Patients having auras scored lower than seizure-free patients on health perceptions, energy/fatigue, role limitations due to emotional problems, cognitive function and role limitations due to memory problems. This concurs with Hermann et al (1989) observation that persistent auras are associated with a poorer emotional outcome and highlights the need for an improved seizure outcome classification. Aura patients score higher than seizure patients on health perception, overall quality of life, emotional well being and role limitation due to physical problems. The health perception scales were the most sensitive to change with mean scores differing significantly across all three seizure classifications.

This instrument represents a significant advance in the assessment of post-operative outcome and, with development, should be able to fulfil its intended purpose of assessing effectiveness of temporal lobe surgery programmes. However, such instruments cannot easily identify why individuals with similar seizure outcome appear to have different QOL outcome. Thus, an HRQL measure containing valid scales capable of identifying particular problems, especially those amenable to non-medical intervention, would also be useful.

Novel Antiepileptic Drugs and HRQL

Psychosocial and quality of life issues have been entirely neglected in the assessment of new AEDs in clinical trials. As a consequence such trials may be insensitive to potentially useful treatment effects which could improve quality of life in these refractory patients. In response to the need for the development of more sensitive methods of assessing the efficacy of novel AEDs we produced an HRQL model (Table 2) containing previously validated measures of general health, social satisfaction, anxiety, depression, happiness, overall mood, self-esteem and mastery and a specifically designed seizure severity scale with patient and carer-based components.

The ictal subscale of the seizure severity scale has previously been shown to possess acceptable reliability (alpha 0.85) and validity (Baker et al 1991). The psychometric properties of the other scales included in the model had not previously been assessed but,

Table 2. Scales included in a HRQL model for epilepsy

Domain	Scale	Authors
Physical	• Seizure frequency • Seizure severity • Nottingham Health Profile • Activities of daily living	• Baker et al (1991) • Hunt et al (1981) • Brown & Tomlinson (1984)
Social	• Social Problems Questionnaire	• Corney & Clare (1985)
Psychological	• Hospital Anxiety & Depression • Affect Balance • Profile of Moods States • Self-esteem • Mastery	• Zigmond & Snaith (1983) • Bradburn (1969) • McNair et al (1981) • Rosenberg (1965) • Pearlin & Schooler (1978)

References in Smith et al (1992)

with the exception of the SPQ, they all appear to be internally consistent (alpha 0.69–0.85) in patients with refractory seizures. The psychological profile obtained using these scales is similar in comparison to that of patients attending an epilepsy clinic (Morrow 1990) and significantly poorer than that of patients whose epilepsy is in remission (Jacoby et al 1992). More direct evidence of discriminant construct validity of the model was indicated by the ability of the scales selected to differentiate between two groups (those electing to continue with lamotrigine and those not electing to continue with lamotrigine) who would be expected to have different levels of psychological well-being (Baker et al 1992a).

In a randomised, controlled study (Smith et al 1992) there were significant reductions, on lamotrigine relative to placebo, in partial and tonic-clonic seizures. However, although 41 patients elected to continue with lamotrigine only 11 experienced at least 50% reduction in total seizures suggesting that other factors influenced their decision. The score on lamotrigine, relative to placebo, was significantly lower for the ictal ($P = 0.017$) and carers ($P = 0.035$) sub-scales of the seizure severity scale and significantly higher for the happiness ($P = 0.003$) and mastery scales ($P = 0.003$) indicating that these scales are capable of detecting potentially useful treatment effects.

Although these preliminary results are encouraging several deficiencies in the initial version of the model are evident. General social variables are not adequately assessed and specific social issues—stigma and discrimination, which may be important determinants of psychopathology in epilepsy (Whitman & Hermann 1989) were not addressed. A measure of adjustment to illness, considered by Fallowfield (1990) to be an integral element of the psychological domain of QOL, was not included. Furthermore neither the overt toxicity nor the subtle psychomotor and cognitive effects of AEDs, and their relevance to psychosocial issues, has been investigated. Conversely some of the scales included do not make independent contributions to the model. Finally although this is a patient-perceived measure, recent literature (Krupinski 1980, Calman 1984) indicates that interpretation of this perception should allow for individual expectation and include a measure of the gap between actual and desired QOL.

A revised version of the model excludes redundant scales and incorporates a previously validated measure of stigma (Hyman 1971) and newly developed measures of Life Fulfilment and Impact of Epilepsy which have promising psychometric properties (Baker et al 1992b).

In summary, this patient-based HRQL model provides a framework for investigating the complex interaction between physical, social and psychological well-being in epilepsy. Some of the scales included may be useful as secondary measures of efficacy which could enhance the sensitivity of trials of novel AEDs and the model is being used to assess the outcome of temporal lobe surgery. Finally the revised version of the model is being used to examine QOL and quality of care in an unselected, community-based population. It is only by developing such measures that we can identify and target the particular deficiencies in the delivery of health care for people with epilepsy.

CONCLUSIONS

Health-related quality of life is now accepted as a relevant indicator of medical outcome. There can be little doubt that this is a complex, multi-dimensional concept best measured from the patients perspective. The next decade should witness an explosion of valid HRQL instruments but, ultimately, a selected minority, with the best psychometric properties, will be in general usage. Satisfactory instruments can be used to measure disability, in individuals or communities, in the allocation of limited health care resources or in the assessment of the efficacy of treatment.

Epilepsy is a chronic, disabling condition which, until recently, has been neglected in the HRQL literature. However promising instruments have been developed which have the potential to measure the disability caused by epilepsy, to improve the assessment of the outcome of temporal lobe surgery and enhance the sensitivity of controlled trials of novel AEDs.

REFERENCES

Abbey A, Andrews F. Modelling the Psychological determinants of life quality. Soc Indicators Res 1985; 16:1–34.

Annegers JF, Hauser WA, Elveback LR. Remission of seizures and relapse in patients with epilepsy. Epilepsia 1977; 20:729–737.

Arntson P, Droge D, Norton R, & Murray E. The perceived psychosocial consequences of having epilepsy. In: Whitman S, Hermann B, eds. Psychopathology in Epilepsy: Social Dimensions. New York: Oxford University Press, 1986:143–161.

Bagley CR. Social Psychology of the Child with Epilepsy. London: Routledge & Kegan Paul, 1971.

Baker GA, Smith DF, Dewey M, et al. The development, validity and reliability of a health-related quality of life model for epilepsy. Epilepsy Res. (in submission).

Baker GA, Jacoby A, Smith D, et al. The development of Life Fulfilment and Adjustment to Epilepsy scales. Seizure 1992b; 1(suppl A).

Baker GA, Smith DF, Dewey M, et al. The development of a seizure severity scale as an outcome measure in epilepsy. Epilepsy Res 1991; 8:245–251.

Batzel LW, Dodrill CB, Fraser RT. Further validation of the WPSI vocational scale: comparisons with other correlates of employment in epilepsy. Epilepsia 1980; 21:235–242.

Betts TA. Depression, anxiety and epilepsy. In: Reynolds EH, Trimble MR, eds. Epilepsy & Psychiatry. Edinburgh, Churchill Livingstone, 1981:60–71.

Calman KC. Quality of Life in cancer patients: a hypothesis, J Med Ethics 1984; 10:124–127.

Chaplin JE, Yepez Lasso R, Shorvon SD, Floyd M. National general practice study of epilepsy: the social and psychological effects of a recent diagnosis of epilepsy. Br Med J 1992; 304:1416–1418.

Chaplin JE, Yepez R, Shorvon SD, Floyd M. A quantitative approach to measuring the social effects of epilepsy. Neuroepidemiol 1990; 9:151–158.

Collings JA. Psychosocial well-being and epilepsy: an empirical study. Epilepsia 1990; 31:418–426.

Commission for the Control of Epilpesy and its Consequences. Plan for nationwide action on epilepsy (DHEW Publication No. NIH 78–276). Washington, DC: US Government Printing Office, 1978.

Craig A, Oxley J. Social aspects of epilepsy. In: Laidlaw J, Richens A, Oxley J, eds. A Textbook of Epilepsy. Edinburgh, Churchill Livingstone, 1988:566–610.

Dansky L, Andermann E, Andermann F. Marriage and fertility in epileptic patients. Epilepsia 1980; 21:261–271.

Dodrill CB, Breyer DN, Diamond MB, et al. Psychosocial problems among adults with epilepsy. Epilepsia 1984a; 25:168–175.

Dodrill CB, Beier R, Ksaparick et al. Psychosocial problems in adults with epilepsy: Comparison of findings from four countries. Epilepsia 1984b; 25:176–183.

Dodrill CB, Batzel L, Queisser HR, Temkin NR. An objective method for the assessment of psychological and social problems among epileptics. Epilepsia 1980; 21:123–135.

Drummond MF. Resource allocation decisions in health care: A role for quality of life assessments. J Chron Dis 1987; 40:605–616.

Earl WL. Job stability and family counseling. Epilepsia 1986; 27:215–219.

Elwes RDC, Marshall J, Beattie A, Newman PK. Epilepsy and employment. A community based survey in an area of high unemployment. J Neurol Neurosurg Psychiat 1991; 54:200–203.

Elwes RDC, Johnson AL, Shorvon SD, Reynolds EH. The prognosis for seizure control in newly diagnosed epilepsy. N Engl J Med 1984; 311:944–947.

Engel GL. The need for a new medical model: a challenge for biomedicine. Science 1977; 196:129–36.

Engel J. Outcome with respect to epileptic seizures. In: Engel J, ed. Surgical treatment of the epilepsies. New York: Raven Press, 1987:553–571.

Fallowfield L. The quality of life: the missing measurement in health care. London, Souvenir Press, 1990.

Goodyer I. The influence of epilepsy on family functioning. In: Hoare P, ed. Epilepsy and the family. Manchester: Sanofi UK Limited, 1988:11–18.

Guyatt GH, Veldhuyzen Van Zanten SJO, Feeney DH, Patrick DL. Measuring quality of life in clinical trials: A taxonomy and review. Can Med Assoc J 1989; 140:1442-pages.

Harrison RM, Taylor DC. Childhood seizures: a 25-year follow-up. Lancet 1976; ii:948–51.

Hauser WA, Kurland LT. The epidemiology of epilepsy in Rochester, Minnesota, 1935 through 1967. Epilepsia 1975; 16:1–66.

Hauser WA. Postscript: How should outcome be determined and reported? In: Engel J, ed. Surgical treatment of the epilepsies. New York: Raven Press, 1987; 573–582.

Hermann BP. Psychopathology in epilepsy and learned helplessness. Medical Hypothesis 1979; 5:723–729.

Hermann BP, Wyler AR, Ackerman B, Rosenthal T. Short-term psychological outcome of anterior temporal lobectomy. J Neurosurg 1989; 71:327–334.

Hermann BP, Dikmen S, Wilensky AJ. Increased psychopathology associated with multiple seizure types: fact or artifact. Epilepsia 1982; 23:587–596.

Hermann BP, Whitman S, Wyler A, et al. Psychosocial predictors of psychopathology in epilepsy. Br J Psych 1990; 156:98–105.

Hermann BP, Whitman S. Psychopathology in epilepsy: a multifactiological model. In: Whitman S, Hermann BP, eds. Psychopathology in Epilepsy: Social Dimensions. New York: Churchill Livingstone, 1986; 5–37.

Hyman MD. The stigma of stroke. Geriatrics 1971; 5:132–141.

Jacoby A, Johnson AL, Chadwick D. The psychosocial outcomes of antiepileptic drug withdrawal. Epilepsia 1992.

Jacoby A. Epilepsy and the quality of everyday life: findings from a study of people with well-controlled epilepsy. Soc Sci Med 1992; 34:657–666.

Kendrick AM, Trimble MR. Patient-perceived quality of life: What is important to the patient with epilepsy? Seizure 1992; 1(suppl A).

Krupinski J. Health and quality of life. Soc Sci Med; 1980:203–211.

Matthews WS, Barabas G, Ferrari M. Emotional concomitants of childhood epilepsy. Epilepsia 1982; 23:671–681.

Meldrum BS, Porter RJ, eds. New anticonvulsant drugs. London: J.Libbey, 1986.

Van Belle G, Temkin N. Design strategies in the clinical evaluation of new antiepileptic drugs. In: Pedley TA, Meldrum BS, eds. Recent Advances in Epilepsy Vol 1. Edinburgh: Churchill Livingstone, 1981:93–111.

Mittan RJ. Fear of seizures. In: Whitman S, Hermann BP, eds. Psychopathology in Epilepsy: Social Dimensions. New York: Oxford University Press, 1986:90–121.

Morrow J. An assessment of an epilepsy clinic. In: Chadwick DW, ed. Quality of life and quality of care in epilepsy. Royal Society of Medicine, Round Table Series No.23, 96–104.

National Institutes of Health Consensus Conference, Surgery for Epilepsy. JAMA 1990; 264:729.

Robertson MM. Depression in patients with epilepsy reconsidered. In: Pedley TA, Meldrum BS, eds. Recent Advances in Epilepsy Vol.4. Edinburgh, Churchill Livingstone, 1987:205–240.

Rodin E, Shapiro H, and Lennox K. Epilepsy and life performance. Rehabilitation Literature 1977; 38: 34–38.

Scambler G, Hopkins A. Social class, epileptic activity, and disadvantage at work. J Epidemiol Comm Health 1980; 34:129–33.

Scambler G. Epilepsy: The experience of illness. London, Tavistock & Routledge 1989.

Schipper H, Clinch J, Powell V. Definitions and conceptual issues. In: Spilker B, ed. Quality of life assessments in clinical trials. New York: Raven Press, 1990:pages.

Smith DF, Baker GA, Dewey M, et al. Seizure frequency, patient perceived seizure severity and the psychosocial consequences of intractable epilepsy. Epil Res 1991b; 9:231–241.

Smith DF, Baker GA, Davies G, et al. Outcomes of add-on treatment with lamotrigine in partial epilepsy. Epilepsia 1993; 34(2):312–322.

Spilker B, ed. Quality of life assessments in clinical trials. New York, Raven Press, 1990.

Tan SY, Bruni J. Cognitive behavioral therapy with adult patients with epilepsy: a controled outcome study. Epilepsia 1986; 27:225–233.

Taylor D. Psychosocial issues. In Engel J. ed Surgical Treatment of the Epilepsies, 2nd Edition New York Ravens Press (1993).

Temkin NR, Davies GR. Stress as a risk factor for seizure among adults with epilepsy. Epilepsia 1984; 25:450–456.

Thayer RE. Measurment of activation through self-report. Psychol Reports 1967; 20:663–678.

Thompson PJ, Oxley JR. Socioeconomic accompaniments of severe epilepsy. Epilepsia 1988; 29:S9–S18.

Toone BK, Wheeler M, Fenwick PBC. Sex hormone changes in male epileptics. Clin Endocrinol 1980; 12:391–395.

Trostle JA, Hauser WA, Sharborough FW. Psychologic and social adjustment to epilepsy in Rochester, Minnesota. Neurology 1989; 39:633–637.

Vickrey BG, Hays RD, Graber J, et al. A health-related quality of life instrument for patients evaluated for epilepsy surgery. Med Care 1992; 30:299–319.

Ware JE, Sherbourne CD. A 36-item short-form health survey (SF-36): I. Conceptual framework and item selection. Med Care 1992; vol:pages.

Webster A, Mawer GE. Seizure frequency and major life events in epilepsy. Epilepsia 1989; 30: 162–67.

Whitman S, Hermann BP. The architecture of research in the epilepsy/psychopatholgy field. Epil Res 1989; 3:93–99.

Wilensky AJ, Ojemann LM, Friel PN et al. Cinromide in epilepsy: a pilot study. Epilepsia 1983; 24: 401–409.

Zielinski JJ. Selected psychiatric and psychological aspects of epilepsy as seen by an epidemiologist. In: Whitman S, Hermann BP, eds. Psychopathology in epilepsy. New York: Oxford University Press,1986:38–65.

EPILOGUE

This workshop was intended to provide answers to the following questions:

(1) Do we need scales for measuring variables related to epilepsy as opposed to just measuring seizure frequency?

   The definition of *scale* being: an instrument to simultaneously measure two or more facets of epilepsy to be used in clinical assessment.

(2) What is the rationale for creating these scales?

   A) To improve assessment of epilepsy

   B) To improve communication of comparisons of outcome

   a) in clinical trials

   b) in clinical practice

(3) Should this conference attempt to develop one or several scales during its session or only for future development scales?

(4) Which types of scales have the highest priority (e.g., should patient perceptions about treatment results be incorporated in a scale? Can degrees of treatment failure be expressed by a scale?)

   Several reasons for developing epilepsy scales emerged from the workshop:
   The reduction in seizures alone does not sufficiently account for patient perceived changes; there is a need for improvement of communication and comparisons; the epilepsies are compound syndromes and there is a need not only to comprehensively summarize Health Status, but also to comprehensively summarize patient perceived Quality of Life. If one looks at specific purposes for indexes at least seven can be identified.

(1) There appears to be need for *a status index* like Jones Diagnostic Criteria for Acute Rheumatic Fever, which could be of assistance as a guideline for a clinician to chose the correct treatment.

(2) There is already *a scale to assess risk of recurrence of seizures* when withdrawal of medication is contemplated.

(3) *A scale* might be developed *to define whether patients with a particular seizure frequency and seizure severity have been "exhaustively treated", "well treated", "moderately well treated" or "insufficiently treated";* this might be considered a scale of intractability.

However, intractability is, in principle, a retrospective statement as it is impossible to predict how the patient will respond to new types of treatment.

(4) *An index* may be developed as a guideline *for when a physician should refer the patient to a specialist.*

(5) *Indexes* can be used *to evaluate the quality of care* offered by a medical facility.

(6) Quantitative assessment can be used *to evaluate the economic impact of epilepsy.*

(7) An algorithm could be developed *for the purpose of educating the uninitiated* about important parameters in epilepsy care.

Considering the various types of scale, the question is what to include and what to leave out. It was suggested that perhaps indexes should be derived from one large pool of collected data according to the specific needs. However, collecting the data for this general pool could be hampered by being an excessive burden on the patient and the physician.

Some indexes gauge the opinion of the patient about his quality of life as influenced by his or her epilepsy. It may be appropriate to develop similar scales that record the opinion of the nearest relatives.

There is a pressing need for some quantitative assessment of epilepsy surgery, so the scope of the scales should not be too restrictive. However, whether the scales used in assessment of surgery and in assessment of antiepileptic drug efficacy need to be independent, requires further consideration.

Some felt it to be important not to develop universal scales. One should have a scale to answer a particular question. Scales that need to be developed to be included in a drug efficacy study are quite different from those that are being used by health planners to determine what is the level of need for certain medical provisions.

There are at least two possible approaches to the development of a system of scales:

(1) first to see what variables should be quantified when assessing people with epilepsy, and subsequently to see what variables should be combined to obtain an index, which facilitates judgment of a category of functions that are considered of importance,

(2) to come from the top down, e.g. "Look, these are the scales that exist, these are the general approaches, while we will critique each of those to see which variables are in there, we can either adopt one of these or select a hybrid approach."

The average time to develop and validate a psychometric scale is ten years, so a top/bottom working line is to be highly recommended. In terms of the existing experience and data, a lot of work has already gone into seizure rating and adverse effects and it would be a mistake to start all over. On the other hand there is very little in the psychosocial field. There is also a need for neuropsychological assessment as part of treatment outcome evaluation. It does seem that the choice of tests is complicated by the great variety of tests available. In fact, however, this is more a question of appearance as many test batteries employ the same subsets. Still if you wish to measure functions of the patient in the area of attention, you can subdivide this area in six or seven dimensions for which roughly fifty different tests are available. To get consensus which tests to use may not be easy, while including many tests may lead to an unacceptable increase in variance.

Feinstein has advocated to bring more scientific rigour to the process of scales development. He coined the term Clinimetrics for a discipline that is concerned with the development of tools for the assessment of clinical treatment indicators and outcome in-dexes. In the workshop on which this book is based the traditional approach towards questions like the assessment of seizure characteristics and treatment characteristics were contrasted with clinimetric techniques. In the preceding chapters we presented the specific issues in detail as well as a synthesis of the discussions during which we defined and resolved some aspects of the problems. Future research is needed to develop additional instruments of high quality that will be useful in clinical practice and research.

H. Meinardi
Roger J. Porter

PARTICIPANTS

A.P. Aldenkamp, Ph.D.
Instituut voor Epilepsiebestrijding
Achterweg 5
2103 SW Heemstede
The Netherlands

G.A. Baker, Ph.D., B.A., M.Clin.Psychol.,
A.F.B.Ps.
Principal Clinical Neuropsychologist
University Department of Neurological
Science
Walton Hospital
Rice Lane
Liverpool L9 1AE
United Kingdom

S. Bostantjopoulou, M.D.
Aristotelian University of Thessaloniki
"G. Papanikolaou" Hospital
Neurological Clinic
57010 Thessaloniki
Greece

D.W. Chadwick, M.A., D.M., F.R.C.P.
Professor of Neurology
University Department of Neurological
Science
Walton Hospital
Rice Lane
Liverpool L9 1AE
United Kingdom

J.A. Cramer, B.S.
Department of Veterans Affairs
Medical Center
950 Campbell Avenue
West Haven, Connecticut 06516, U.S.A.

J.S. Duncan, M.A., D.M., M.R.C.P.
Institute of Neurology
National Hospital
Queen Square, London WC1N 3BG
United Kingdom

A.R. Feinstein, M.S., M.D.
Sterling Professor of Medicine and
Epidemiology
Clinical Epidemiology Unit
Yale University Medical School
333 Cedar Street - I 456 SHM
P.O. Box 3333
New Haven, Connecticut 06510, U.S.A.

Y.A. Hekster, Ph.D.
Department of Clinical Pharmacy
University Hospital Nijmegen
P.O. Box 9101
6500 HB Nijmegen
The Netherlands

P. Jallon, M.D.
Privat-Dozent
Chief, EEG Department
Hôpital Cantonal Universitaire de Genève
24 rue Micheli-du-Crest
CH-1211 Genève 14
Switzerland

A.L. Johnson, Ph.D., CStat.
Medical Statistician
MRC Biostatistics Unit
Institute of Public Health
University Forvie Site
Robinson Way
Cambridge CB2 2SR
United Kingdom

D.G.A. Kasteleijn-Nolst Trenité, M.D.
Chief, Research Support Unit
Instituut voor Epilepsiebestrijding
P.O. Box 21
2100 AA Heemstede
The Netherlands

A. Kazis, M.D.
Aristotelian University of Thessaloniki
"G. Papanikolaou" Hospital
Neurological Clinic
57010 Thessaloniki
Greece

A. Keyser, M.D., Ph.D.
Department of Neurology
St. Radboud Ziekenhuis
P.O. Box 9101
6500 HB Nijmegen
The Netherlands

M.W. Lammers, M.D.
Department of Neurology
St. Radboud Ziekenhuis
P.O. Box 9101
6500 HB Nijmegen
The Netherlands

A. Martins da Silva, M.D., Ph.D.
Serviço de Neurofisiologia
Hospital Geral de Santo António
4000 Porto
Portugal

R.H. Mattson, M.D.
Neurology Service - 127
Department of Veterans Affairs
Medical Center
950 Campbell Avenue
West Haven, Connecticut 06516, U.S.A.

H. Meinardi, M.D., Ph.D.
Instituut voor Epilepsiebestrijding
P.O. Box 21
2100 AA Heemstede
The Netherlands

D. Mendonça, Ph.D.
Instituto de Ciências Biomédicas de Abel
Salazar
Universidade do Porto
Largo Prof. Abel Salazar 2
4000 Porto
Portugal

Belina Nunez, M.D.
Neurologist
Serviço de Neurofisiologia
Hospital Geral Santo António
4000 Porto
Portugal

B. Pedersen, M.D.
Head, Department of Neurology
Aalborg Sygenhus Syd
DK-9100 Aalborg
Denmark

R.J. Porter, M.D.
Vice President, Clinical Pharmacology
Wyeth-Ayerst Research
145 King of Prussia Road
Radnor, Pennsylvania 19087, USA

W.O. Renier, M.D., Ph.D.
Lecturer in Epileptology
Interdisciplinary Child Neurology Center
University Hospital
P.O. Box 9101
6500 HB Nijmegen
The Netherlands

B. Spilker, M.D., Ph.D.
Orphan Medical
13911 Ridgedale Drive
Minnetonka, Minnesota 55305, U.S.A.

J. Vermeulen, D.Psychol.
Neuropsychologist
Instituut voor Epilepsiebestrijding
Achterweg 5
2103 SW Heemstede
The Netherlands

C. Viteri, M.D.
Departamento de Neurología
Clínica Universitaria
Avda. Pío XII, 36
31080 Pamplona
Spain

AUTHOR INDEX

SUBJECT INDEX